TRAUMATIC BRAIN INJURY
IN CHILDREN AND ADOLESCENTS

The Guilford School Practitioner Series

EDITORS

STEPHEN N. ELLIOTT, PhD
University of Wisconsin–Madison

JOSEPH C. WITT, PhD
Louisiana State University, Baton Rouge

Recent Volumes

Traumatic Brain Injury in Children and Adolescents:
Assessment and Intervention
MARGARET SEMRUD-CLIKEMAN

Schools and Families: Creating Essential Connections for Learning
SANDRA L. CHRISTENSON and SUSAN M. SHERIDAN

Homework Success for Children with ADHD:
A Family–School Intervention Program
THOMAS J. POWER, JAMES L. KARUSTIS, and DINA F. HABBOUSHE

Conducting School-Based Assessments of Child and Adolescent Behavior
EDWARD S. SHAPIRO and THOMAS R. KRATOCHWILL, Editors

Designing Preschool Interventions: A Practitioner's Guide
DAVID W. BARNETT, SUSAN H. BELL, and KAREN T. CAREY

Effective School Interventions
NATALIE RATHVON

DSM-IV Diagnosis in the Schools
ALVIN E. HOUSE

Medications for School-Age Children: Effects on Learning and Behavior
RONALD T. BROWN and MICHAEL G. SAWYER

Advanced Applications of Curriculum-Based Measurement
MARK R. SHINN, Editor

Brief Intervention for School Problems: Collaborating for Practical Solutions
JOHN J. MURPHY and BARRY L. DUNCAN

Academic Skills Problems: Direct Assessment and Intervention, Second Edition
EDWARD S. SHAPIRO

Social Problem Solving: Interventions in the Schools
MAURICE J. ELIAS and STEVEN E. TOBIAS

Instructional Consultation Teams: Collaborating for Change
SYLVIA A. ROSENFIELD and TODD A. GRAVOIS

Traumatic Brain Injury
in Children and Adolescents

ASSESSMENT AND INTERVENTION

◆ ◆ ◆

Margaret Semrud-Clikeman

◆

THE GUILFORD PRESS
New York   London

© 2001 The Guilford Press
A Division of Guilford Publications, Inc.
72 Spring Street, New York, NY 10012
www.guilford.com

Printed in the United States of America

This book is printed on acid-free paper.

Last digit is print number: 9   8   7   6   5   4   3   2   1

Library of Congress Cataloging-in-Publication Data

Semrud-Clikeman, Margaret.
   Traumatic brain injury in children and adolescents : assessment and
intervention / Margaret Semrud-Clikeman.
      p.   cm. — (The Guilford school practitioner series)
   Includes bibliographical references and index.
   ISBN 1-57230-686-6 (hard)
   1. Brain-damaged children—Rehabilitation. 2. Brain—Wounds and
injuries—Patients—Rehabilitation. 3. Brain—Wounds and injuries—
Complications. I. Title. II. Series.
   [DNLM: 1. Brain Injuries—diagnosis—Adolescence. 2. Brain
Injuries—diagnosis—Child. 3. Brain Injuries—therapy—
Adolescence. 4. Brain Injuries—therapy—Child. WS 340 S473t 2001]
   RC496.B7 S458 2001
   617.4'81044'083—dc21

                                                      2001023143

*This book is dedicated to the many children
and their families with whom I have had
the privilege to work.*

*It is also dedicated to my family.
In particular, I would like to mention the support
of my father, Ray Semrud,
and my husband, John Clikeman.*

About the Author

♦

Margaret Semrud-Clikeman, PhD, is Associate Professor of Educational Psychology at the University of Texas at Austin. She received her master's degree from the University of Wisconsin–Madison and her PhD from the University of Georgia. Dr. Semrud-Clikeman was a school psychologist in Wisconsin for 13 years prior to beginning her doctoral education. She completed a neuroscience fellowship at Massachusetts General Hospital/ McLean Hospital/Harvard Medical School and received the early career award from the National Academy of Neuropsychology in 1999 for her contributions in clinical neuropsychology. Dr. Semrud-Clikeman's current interests include the neuroanatomical and neuropsychological underpinnings of attention-deficit/hyperactivity disorder and developmental disorders, interventions, and issues in the training of school psychologists.

Preface

◆

This book serves as a guide to traumatic brain injury (TBI) for school psychologists, clinical child psychologists, and educators. It was written for professionals who are not neuropsychologists and who have little training in the field, and provides an understanding of the underpinnings of head injury, beginning with definitions, incidence, and sequelae. Throughout the volume I present examples that are a combination of the many cases with whom I have worked over the past 25 years. These composites make the material "come alive" for the professional and illustrate the typical child or adolescent that the school professional or private clinician may see over the course of his/her experience.

The book is organized to provide basic information as well as a brief summary of neuroanatomy as a background for understanding the ramifications of TBI. Since most clinicians and school personnel do not see the child in the initial stages of recovery, it is very important to understand the "language" used by medical personnel in order to provide appropriate programming for the child/adolescent once he/she returns to school. Thus, the middle part of the book provides an overview of the most commonly utilized instruments that comprise a neuropsychological assessment. The administration and interpretation of evaluation tools used by school psychologists and clinical child psychologists in the assessment of children with TBI are covered in this section.

One area that has not been given the attention it merits is the contribution of family variables to the recovery of children with TBI. Family cohesion has been found to be an important aspect of a child's eventual recovery. School psychologists and educators have a responsibility to assist the family in the child's reentry into school. In addition and most important, it is imperative that the school and family form a partnership to assist with this reentry and in the ensuing years of school. Thus, a chapter is devoted

ix

to the family, with recommendations to facilitate the forming of school–home collaboration.

The third section of this volume is devoted to developing appropriate interventions for the child within the school setting. This section was one of the more difficult to write, as there are few studies documenting the efficacy of interventions over time for children with TBI. As such, interventions were borrowed from the fields of attention-deficit/hyperactivity disorder and learning disabilities as well as from the field of adult rehabilitation.

Finally, a composite case history, using data derived from three representative cases, is used to illustrate a child's recovery from TBI. This composite will assist school personnel in understanding the course of recovery from TBI and the support they can provide with this process.

Having worked with children with all types of disabilities over the past 25 years, I know first-hand the concerns that school personnel have for these students. One of my goals in writing this volume was to provide information that school practitioners can use in their work with these children. I hope that together we will continue to advance our knowledge of their needs and of appropriate interventions for their recovery.

In closing, I would like to acknowledge the help that I received from the two reviewers of this book, Mike Havey and Laurie G. Dodge. Their suggestions and help were invaluable in the preparation of this volume.

Contents

◆

CHAPTER 1

♦♦♦

Introduction

♦

Richard reluctantly entered my office accompanied by his concerned mother. This 16-year-old male was recovering from an encounter with a tree that he hit head-on in his car. Richard had just been discharged from a rehabilitation hospital after a 3-month stay and was scheduled to rejoin his junior class the following week. He suffered major trauma to his frontal and temporal lobes as well as a skull fracture. He was in a coma for 3 days after the accident and was in intensive physical and occupational therapy since regaining consciousness. He has received homebound instruction at the hospital for the past 3 months and has made good progress. Prior to the accident Richard was an honor student with a 3.75 grade point average. Although his achievement levels continued to be on target for his grade placement, Richard was experiencing significant problems with learning and retaining new material. His prognosis for recovery was guarded. Richard's frustration level was high, and his mother reported that he had become more labile since the accident. Moreover, Richard denied that he was experiencing any difficulty and angrily refuted his mother's statements about his learning problems. As a school psychologist and pediatric neuropsychologist, I was asked by the school system to evaluate Richard and to assist in the development of an Individualized Education Plan (IEP).

My interview with Richard confirmed his mother's report that he would not acknowledge any difficulty. His mother was very concerned and repeatedly asked whether Richard would ever attain the level of academic achievement seen prior to the accident. She also expressed some anger at Richard because he had not worn his seatbelt and had been overconfident in his driving the car.

This case exemplifies the problems present when children and adolescents return to school following a traumatic brain injury (TBI). There are not only neuropsychological and educational issues that need to be addressed, there are also emotional and familial issues that must be evaluated. Prior to the accident, Richard had been a high-functioning adolescent who had individuated from his family and was fairly independent. Following the accident, not only did Richard show neuropsychological deficits, he had also returned to a dependent relationship with his parents. Understandably, Richard's parents had become very protective of their son. The school needed to provide a program for Richard that met his educational, emotional, and social needs. The challenge I faced was to assist in devising this plan while also assisting his family in understanding Richard's new level of functioning. Yet before we could get to that point, the family needed to go through some grieving over the loss of the preaccident Richard.

The aim of this book is to provide school and private clinicians with a knowledge base of traumatic brain injury (TBI) from a transactional viewpoint. Such a viewpoint takes into consideration the interaction of many variables in TBI, including the underlying neuropsychological deficits and the educational, social, and family needs in developing a program for children and adolescents recovering from TBI. Each of these systems (school, peers, and family) interact with the disorder and either assist or hinder the child's recovery. Because the purpose of this book is to provide practical guidance and knowledge of TBI, the rest of the text addresses issues related to the assessment, diagnosis, and treatment of TBI. Thus, the following chapters include a brief summary of functional neuroanatomy, the neuropsychological correlates of TBI, generally accepted assessment practices, family issues, and an overview of interventions.

DEFINITIONS

A head injury can be either closed or open. An *open-head injury* generally involves a wound caused by a missile (i.e., bullet) or some other type of open wound. Such injuries, which are rarer than closed-head injuries, are not addressed in this book. A *closed-head injury* to a child is caused by the child's head striking a hard surface, falling, or experiencing abuse (shaken baby syndrome). Head trauma is generally the result of acceleration/deceleration forces with or without impact of the skull (Bruce, 1990). Seizures are seen after head trauma in approximately 3–5% of children. These seizures frequently occur in the first 24 hours after the trauma (Bruce, 1990).

Two types of injuries are generally seen with closed-head injury: focal and diffuse. *Focal injury* results from impact and is associated with a skull fracture or brain contusion. This type of injury is generally seen in falls from bicycles. The impact of the head on a stationary structure results in the injury. When this impact occurs, there is damage at the point of impact and at the region involved in the rebound from the impact. The original impact is termed the *coup*, and the rebound blow is the *contrecoup*. A contrecoup involves the impact of the brain on the area of the skull opposite to the point of original impact, causing a bruise or hematoma. Both of these impact points serve as localizers for the assessment of damage (Lezak, 1994). Thus, hitting one's head in the front may also cause damage in the posterior of the brain.

Diffuse injury is the result of the shearing of white matter and gray matter due to the acceleration/deceleration of the brain. This damage is generally caused by the stretching and distortion of the axons (see Chapter 2), and such neuronal disruption often results in a coma. Diffuse injury is most commonly seen in the structures that are involved in the transfer of information from one hemisphere to the other (corpus callosum), from tracts running from anterior to posterior regions (internal capsule), and in structures responsible for balance and skilled movements (cerebellum). In addition, damage is frequently seen in the region of the frontal lobes in the area of the eye sockets and in the regions in front of the ears (the temporal poles). Damage to these areas has been found to influence behavior, emotion, memory, and attention. Diffuse injury is most frequently seen with car accidents and child abuse.

Injury due to an accident itself, whether focal or diffuse, is considered a *primary effect*. *Secondary effects* are those that result from the original injury and affect recovery. Secondary effects that increase the likelihood of additional damage include brain swelling, areas of ischemia (death of neurons), contusions of the brain, tearing or shearing of the white matter of the brain, hemorrhage, and subdural hematomas (Graham et al., 1989a, 1989b). Follow-up studies of children after head injury utilizing magnetic resonance imaging (MRI) have found a 50% incidence of bruising (contusions) of the frontal and/or temporal cortex (Levin et al., 1993; Mendelson et al., 1992). Moreover, additional follow-up studies of children with moderate to severe TBI have found poor cognitive skills despite normal MRI scans (Levin et al., 1993). This finding makes it crucial for school and clinical professionals to be alert to lack of progress or deterioration of skills even after a clean bill of health has been provided by medical professionals. Repeat MRI or computed tomography (CT) scanning has been found to identify lesions that initially could not be seen (Levin et al., 1993).

SEVERITY

There are variations in the severity of head injury, ranging from mild, to moderate, to severe. The Glasgow Coma Scale (GCS; Jennett & Teasdale, 1981) is frequently used to ascertain the level of head injury. This scale, which evaluates the child's level of consciousness and response, includes a number of categories: death, persistent vegetative state, severe disability, moderate disability, and good recovery. It assesses eye opening (spontaneous to no eye opening), motor responses, and verbal responses and ranges from a score of 3 to 15. The higher the score, the less impairment is present. The GSC has been validated extensively with adults but has been reported to show less reliability for young, preverbal children (Lehr, 1990). Table 1.1 presents the behaviors assessed by the GCS.

The duration of impaired consciousness—that is, the number of days from the time of injury until the child is able to follow commands—is used to gauge the severity of head trauma. Severe injuries are generally seen when impaired consciousness exceeds 24 hours. The highest rates of fatality are for those patients with a GCS score of 8 or less (Henry et al., 1992; Luerssen et al., 1988; Wagstyl et al., 1987).

The Children's Coma Scale was designed for children under the age of 3 (Raimondi & Hirschauer, 1984). Unfortunately, there have been few studies to validate this scale and its predictive validity is unknown. It allows for the assessment of eye movement rather than response to commands, to nonverbal reactions (crying and breathing rate) rather than talking, and basic motor movements (flexion and extension) rather than motor responses to commands.

TABLE 1.1. Glasgow Coma Scale

Behavior	Points
Eye opening (E)	
Spontaneous	4
In response to speech	3
In response to pinprick (pain)	2
No response	1
Motor (M)	
Follows commands	6
Can localize pain	5
Withdraws from painful stimulus	4
Abnormal flexion to pain	3
Extensor response to pain	2
No response	1
Verbal (V)	
Oriented	5
Confused conversation	4
Inappropriate words	3
Incomprehensible sounds	2
No response	1

Note. Coma score = E + M + V. Data from Jennett and Teasdale (1981).

The length of posttraumatic amnesia (PTA)—the time required for the child to be able to understand time and spatial orientation and to recall prior events—is another measure of the severity of injury. The length of PTA has been found to correlate with impaired reading ability in those with severe injury. A PTA of more than 1 week shows the greatest degree of reading impairment, with some improvement seen over time (Chadwick et al., 1981a). Other investigators have found that closed-head injury is related to deficits in language, with severe closed-head injury more typically related to significant impairment than mild closed-head injury (Ewing-Cobbs et al., 1987). When the duration of the coma state was evaluated for resulting deficits 1 year posttrauma, Ruijs and colleagues (1990) found that children in longer comas showed more behavioral changes, more school problems, and more neuropsychological deficits than those with shorter comas. Bruce (1990) suggests that up to 50% of children who recover consciousness after severe head trauma and loss of consciousness for more than 6 hours will show some intellectual and/or psychiatric problems in the first 2 years after the trauma.

Mild Head Injury

Mild head injury constitutes approximately 50–75% of all traumatic head injuries (Frankowski et al., 1985). Many of these are not fully evaluated by medical personnel or are dismissed as nonremarkable (Doronzo, 1990). Mild head injury is difficult to assess (Lustig & Thompkins, 1998). Meta-analytic studies have indicated that definitions of mild head injury vary from a bump on the head to a concussion. Without a consensus about the definition of such an injury, the findings of various studies are equivocal.

Mild head injuries are those that result in a loss of consciousness or PTA of less than 1 hour and a GCS score of 13 to 15. Throughout their development, many children have minor blows to the head that are not considered problematic by most clinicians (National Head Injury Foundation, 1985). Begali (1992) suggests that even lesser concussions can produce some minor damage to brain stem nuclei. Concussions have generally been assumed to have few ramifications for later functioning. However, emerging evidence suggests that there may be some damage to the reticular activating system in the brainstem (allows for arousal and attention), as well as in the cerebral hemispheres (Jane & Rimel, 1982; Levin et al., 1982; Pang, 1985). There is also some evidence indicating that repeated blows to the head may be cumulative, with the rate of recovery being lengthened with each concussion (Binder & Rattok, 1989). Soccer players who hit the ball repeatedly with the head have been found to achieve lower scores on neuropsychological measures (Witol & Webbe, 1994); the poorest scores are found for children who played the most games (Abreau et al., 1990). Particular weaknesses were found on measures of attention and information processing. These findings have been replicated in professional soccer players, who were found to show mild to moderate neuropsychological impairment, with documented cerebral atrophy in one-third of the sample (Tysvaer, 1992; Tysvaer et al., 1989).

Findings in cases of mild head injury indicate that most children and adolescents are conscious when they enter the emergency room of a hospital and present with normal neurological findings (Friedman, 1983; Levin et al., 1982). Mild head injuries may be accompanied by headache, lethargy, irritability, withdrawal, and/or lability (Begali, 1992; Boll, 1982). Such behavioral changes can persist and result in difficulties in school and within the family unit (Boll, 1983). Children under the age of 12 with minor head injuries have been found to show behavioral difficulties such as attentional deficit and low frustration tolerance even 4 years postinjury (Klonoff et al., 1977). Changes in IQ are very infrequent in children with mild TBI, although subtle complex language deficits and attention difficulties may be present for 6 months or longer after the injury has occurred. The most affected area of neuropsychological functioning is the ability of the child to comprehend language and process incoming verbal information (Begali, 1992). Thus, information processing difficulties constitute the most common type of deficit and may partially explain the higher-than-expected number of children with minor head injury prior to age 12 being retained in a grade or being placed in remedial classes (Alves & Jane, 1985; Boll, 1983; Ylvisaker, 1985).

Bijur and colleagues (1990) found a significant relationship between mild head injury and hyperactivity in a large sample of children. Similarly, a major study on mild closed-head injury compared children with mild TBI, children with other injuries, and control children (Asarnow et al., 1995). It was found that although children/adolescents with mild head injury showed an increased number of behavioral problems, many of these children had had behavioral problems *prior* to the accident. This finding is supportive of previous hypotheses that children with more behavioral problems are at heightened risk for accidents and TBI (Brown et al., 1981).

Asarnow and colleagues (1995) compared a group of children with mild TBI, children with injury other than head trauma, and a control group on a series of behavioral and neuropsychological measures. Behavioral problems were found in both the TBI group and the other injury group as compared with controls. These deficits in functioning were present 12 months postinjury. During this 12-month period, behaviors were found to have improved in both injury groups. In support of this finding, Donders (1992) found that the rate of premorbid psychological and behavioral difficulties in children who later experience TBI is similar to the rate in the general pediatric population. In contrast, children with severe TBI show increased behavioral difficulties following their injuries (Asarnow et al., 1991).

Asarnow and colleagues (1995) did not find significant neuropsychological impairment in children with mild TBI in the areas of academic performance and information processing. No differences were found on measures of receptive language, executive functioning, and motor skills. Difficulty was found in the mild TBI group on measures of memory, with attentional deficits approaching significance ($p = .06$). Moreover, both injury groups (head injury and other injury) scored more poorly on the attention and memory tasks. The authors concluded that, *irrespective* of the type of injury, the experience of having an injury and the stress it involves may result in nonspecific memory difficulties, which appear to resolve with time. Asarnow and colleagues suggest that children who have a period of unconsciousness of less than 30 minutes and whose PTA is also less than 30 minutes do not show significant functional morbidity following recovery.

These findings are inconsistent with earlier findings suggesting that even mild head injury can cause significant behavioral deficits. One of the differences in the aforementioned study is that evidence of premorbid functioning was obtained for the sample and indicated that these children had behavioral and learning difficulties *prior* to their accidents. Although the accidents did produce transient symptoms, these symptoms were not present 1 year after the injuries.

Bijur and Haslum (1995) suggest that the persistent deficits seen in mild TBI are subtler and show greater variability than those seen in severe TBI. These investigators utilized a sample taken from a study of 12,000 children born in Britain during a 1-week period in 1970, who were studied at ages 5 and 10. In this sample 112 children had experienced mild head injuries requiring outpatient or hospital treatment. These children were compared with another subsample from the British cohort who had no injuries and others who had limb fractures or lacerations. There was no difference in intellectual achievement between the head-injured and control groups. Slightly lower scores, although not significantly different, were found for the head-injured group in reading and mathematics achievement. Some difficulty was found in hyperactivity, but differences between groups did not continue when demographic variables were covaried.

The conclusion from this large-scale study was similar to that of Asarnow and colleagues (1995), namely, that little evidence of long-term cognitive difficulties was found in children with mild head injury. However, behavioral difficulties were noted, and as suggested by the studies discussed earlier, it is likely that premorbid behavioral difficulties are related to a tendency toward TBI and that these difficulties continue, or possibly worsen, following an accident. Thus, the impact of minor TBI is unknown at this time. The school psychologist and clinical psychologist must take these concerns into account and must be aware that careful monitoring of children returning to school after mild TBI is crucial for appropriate programming.

Moderate Head Injury

When loss of consciousness or PTA lasts from 1 to 24 hours and the GCS score is 9 to 12, the injury is considered to be moderate. Symptoms that appear to persist over time include headache, memory deficits, and behavioral difficulties. These symptoms tend to persist for several months, and, similar to those with mild TBI, many patients with moderate TBI have a history of previous head injuries (Naugle, 1990). For these patients, secondary symptoms are more common, including hematomas and edema (brain swelling) that require surgery. Deficits are frequently found on neuropsychological measures, particularly in the areas of problem solving, memory, and attention/concentration (Rimel et al., 1982). Because of these problems, many patients with moderate head injuries experience difficulty in caring for their needs and, for adults, in maintaining employment.

Children with moderate head injuries have been found to resemble those with mild head injuries, in terms of sequelae, more than those with severe head injuries (Levin et al., 1988). In fact, the research generally combines mildly and moderately head-injured children into one group, making it difficult to ascertain individual functioning (Asarnow et al., 1995). Many of the studies of mild TBI have incorporated children with PTA and loss of consciousness that is more severe than most would consider "mild" (Ewing-Cobbs et al., 1989; Mahalick, 1990). Thus, our knowledge of mild and moderate head injury is in its infancy, and like mildly head-injured patients, those with moderate injury should be carefully monitored and serially evaluated for progress. Of 30 articles reviewed by Asarnow and colleagues (1995) from 1971 to 1993, only 11 included groups with moderate head injury and 3 included the moderate with the mild group. Thus, more than 50% of the articles did not include a moderate head injury group.

Severe Head Injury

Injuries that result in a loss of consciousness or PTA for more than 24 hours with a GCS of 3 to 8 are considered to be severe (Begali, 1992). Patients with these injuries frequently require immediate and intensive medical treatment. Approximately 50% of children brought to an emergency room with severe head injuries die (Fletcher et al., 1995). For those who survive, the deficits are more severe, both physically and neuropsychologically, than those of children with mild to moderate head injury. The hospital stay is longer, and these children are twice as likely to suffer additional injuries (broken limbs, etc.). Most children with severe injury are found to have been pedestrians in a traffic accident or passengers in a motor vehicle accident, whereas those with mild injuries are generally injured during play (Asarnow et al., 1995).

Upon recovery, many severely injured children and adolescents show intellectual impairment that does not resolve as well as psychiatric difficulties. Achievement in school is often significantly compromised by deficits in the ability to name objects and/or pictures, in verbal fluency, and in the ability to take written notes; children are typically more impaired than adolescents (Ewing-Cobbs et al., 1986, 1991). Additional deficits in memory, attention, and organization have repeatedly been found in children with severe head injuries (Jaffe et al., 1985). The length of coma has been found to be associated with enduring cognitive impairment and the inability to return to school, with longer comas associated with poorer outcomes (Ruff et al., 1990, 1993).

For adults, recovery from head injury is usually completed within 180 days of injury, with as much recovery as will be achieved almost always present within 6 to 9 months of injury (Lezak, 1994). For children, recovery from severe TBI can span 5 to 6 years postinjury (Beaumont, 1983; Luria, 1963). However, the first 12 to 18 months after coma is considered the most crucial period for recovery, as 85% of all cognitive and behavioral improvement is found in that period. Some children show significant improvements 2 to 3 years after injury (Barth & Macciocchi, 1985; Rutter et al., 1983).

Green and colleagues (1998) studied children with moderate to severe TBI for emotional functioning following their injuries. All children were assessed at approximately the same amount of time from the original injury. The Achenbach Child Behavior Checklist (CBCL; Achenbach, 1991), Personality Inventory for Children (PIC; Lachar, Kline, & Boersma, 1986), and psychiatric interviews were administered to each child and parent. There was a significant discrepancy between the rating scales and the interviews, in that the rating scales showed a low rate of psychological disturbance and the interviews showed a high rate. It was suggested that the rating scales may not have been sensitive to a child's impairment because of the forced-choice format, whereas the interviews provided an opportunity for the parent to expand and elaborate responses. The highest rate of disorder was found for anxiety, based on the interviews, and attentional problems were highlighted on the CBCL. It was recommended, based on the results of this study, that structured clinical interviews may be the most appropriate means of determining whether patients meet the criteria for various diagnoses and that the CBCL is most helpful in evaluating difficulty with attention and impulse control, but not for diagnosis.

Shaffer (1995) conducted a comprehensive evaluation of children with mild and severe head injury. For those children with severe TBI, the rate of psychiatric disorder appearing directly after injury was higher and was present in children without neurological abnormality or intellectual impairment to a greater degree than in the other groups (control, mild TBI). Preinjury behavior was found to be the most powerful predictor for later problems in all of the groups. Of the children with severe TBI, 61.9% were found to evidence a new psychiatric disorder within 2 years of the injury, as compared with 20% of the children with mild TBI and 13.6 % of the controls. The majority of the children with severe TBI were found to show disinhibition and socially inappropriate behavior.

These behaviors are reminiscent of attention-deficit/hyperactivity disorder (ADHD), and in two of Shaffer's cases ADHD evolved after recovery. These difficulties have been linked to frontal lobe dysfunction in studies with adults and with primates (Lezak, 1994; Luria, 1963). Moreover, research using MRI correlates in ADHD have implicated the frontal lobe, particularly the right frontal white matter (Filipek et al., 1998; Semrud-Clikeman et al., 2000).

The conclusion drawn from Shaffer's study (1995) was that TBI may not be an all-or-none effect—that psychiatric comorbidity is present and is most common in those children who have a history of behavioral difficulties and who come from poor psychosocial environments. Shaffer also found central nervous system damage to be the most powerful risk factor for later development of psychiatric disorders in children, a finding substantiated by other studies (e.g., Teeter & Semrud-Clikeman, 1997). The most disturbing finding of Shaffer's work is that support services for children with such psychiatric disturbances were not routinely implemented and frequently not provided.

DEMOGRAPHICS

Incidence

The incidence of children and adolescents experiencing TBI has increased, and head injury has become the leading cause of death in those under age 35. Children under 15 years of age with head injuries account for more than half of all deaths due to trauma (Fletcher et al., 1995). This incidence is significantly higher than the incidence of childhood deaths resulting from the second leading cause, childhood leukemia. Kraus (1995) reports that in cases of head injury, for each death resulting from a head injury, there were 32 hospital discharges and 152 children who were medically attended in 1991. Among those children who did not die from their injuries, a significant proportion had learning and behavioral difficulties.

Of those children with severe TBI, 80% have been found to have particular educational needs or to require modified educational environments 2 years postinjury (Ewing-Cobbs et al., 1991). Behavioral difficulties are also relatively prevalent even among those children with mild head injuries (Fletcher et al., 1995). The majority of children admitted alive to the hospital are discharged with a prognosis for good recovery. However, good recovery does not mean full recovery, and many of the children have been later found to evidence temporary to permanent difficulties in cognition, memory, or physical disability (Jennett & Teasdale, 1981; Kraus, 1995).

Risk Factors

Males are more prone to have head injuries than females by an almost 2:1 ratio, particularly when the children are aged 5 to 14 (Kraus, 1995). Prior to age 5 the ratio of males to females is fairly even. Age is a second factor that contributes to TBI. Prior to age 5 the incidence of head injury is lower than after age 5, with the increase most pronounced for males. The rates for females decline in late childhood (Kraus, 1995).

Children in special education classes for behavioral disorders have been found to have a threefold likelihood of previous head injury, as compared with those in regular education (Michaud et al., 1993). Children in special education were compared with children in regular education classes as to the prevalence of head injuries. A history of preschool head injury was more than seven times more frequent in children in special education than in the control group. Thus, Kraus (1995) suggests that children with brain injury of any severity be followed over time to determine the presence or degree of cognitive or behavioral difficulty.

Children with ADHD have also been found to be at higher risk for head injury, possibly due to their impulsive behaviors and inattention (Teeter & Semrud-Clikeman, 1997). In addition, children who experience brain injury have been found to differ from the noninjured population in several ways. They tended to have higher rates of premorbid behavioral difficulties (Asarnow et al., 1995; Donders, 1992) and more temperamental and family difficulties (Bijur et al., 1990; Bijur & Haslum, 1995) than children who experienced no brain injury. For example, a longitudinal study by Bijur and colleagues (1990, 1995) found that children with TBI more frequently showed aggression and hyperactivity prior to the injuries and had mothers with higher depression scores than those of the control group.

Age and Developmental Factors

The age of the child has been found to be closely related to the type of injury sustained. For infants and toddlers the most common cause of head trauma is a fall, with few long-term consequences. Severe head trauma at this age is generally due to child abuse or automobile injury. For young children through elementary school the most common causes of head injury are pedestrian and bicycle accidents. For teenagers injury is generally due to automobile accidents in which the teenager is the driver (Bruce, 1990). When multiple traumas occur, the prognosis is significantly poorer (Luerssen et al., 1988).

Age is an important variable in understanding the sequelae of TBI. Younger children show different patterns of recovery, and future learning is further affected because of their incomplete development (Brazelli et al., 1994; Johnson, 1992; Teeter & Semrud-Clikeman, 1997). Early injury has been found to be related to more significant later deficits than later injury (Teeter, 1986). The developing brain may be more vulnerable to damage because of the rapid growth spurts that occur in the early stages. Kolb and Whishaw (1990) suggest three critical age divisions influencing the prognosis of a child with TBI: (1) less than 1 year of age, (2) between 1 and 5 years of age, and (3) more than 5 years of age. Damage occurring prior to age 1 appears to result in significant impairment, whereas damage between ages 1 and 5 allows for the reorganization of functions and recovery of language ability. Damage occurring after age 5, again, is quite significant and may impair the normal process of brain development (O'Leary & Boll, 1984).

Structures that do not generally develop until later in life may be compromised by early damage, and this injury may not be obvious until years later (Rourke et al., 1983). Particularly vulnerable to this condition are tasks that involve frontal lobe and association areas of the brain—these areas do not assume adult-like functions until 12 years of age or later (Teeter & Semrud-Clikeman, 1997). Frontal lobe tasks generally measure the ability to monitor behavior and allow a person to change behavior according to the situation, and association areas allow for the integration of information from various modalities (visual–motor, visual–spatial, auditory–visual, etc.).

Levin and colleagues (1995) found that children with severe head injury are more likely to continue to show intellectual impairment, as compared with adolescents with the same extent of damage. In preschoolers, intellectual ability was found to be related to severity of head injury, with those with mild to moderate injury showing more intellectual improvement (Ewing-Cobbs et al., 1989). Expressive language skills were found to be more susceptible to early TBI than receptive language (Ewing-Cobbs et al., 1987).

Young children experiencing TBI in infancy were found to have more receptive and expressive language problems than those with TBI as toddlers (Ewing-Cobbs et al., 1989). In addition, preadolescents with TBI were found to have less improvement in writing than older adolescents with TBI (Ewing-Cobbs et al., 1987). Similarly, recovery in motor and visual–spatial tasks was found to be slower in younger adolescents than in older adolescents (Thompson et al., 1994). Johnson (1992) found that children with TBI continued to show memory and language deficits even after successful school reentry. Moreover, these children were found to show severe learning difficulties years after the injury, which were not initially apparent.

MEDICAL ASSESSMENT

Prior to the current development of the advanced technology involved in MRI and CT scans, autopsies provided much of the evidence for brain damage. With the advent of these technologies it is now possible to obtain *in vivo* pictures and to begin to ascertain the effects of TBI and its relationship to various neuropsychological deficits. MRI and CT scans allow for the evaluation of compromised structures of the brain and are often utilized in initial assessment. Some neuropsychological deficits have been found in children with TBI with normal MRI scans, possibly indicating that there are differences in cerebral blood flow that cannot be seen in structural MRI scans but which, nevertheless, produce symptoms. An assessment for TBI generally involves the use of the GCS, a good medical history and examination, and the use of MRI and/or CT scans.

CT scans use a narrow X-ray beam that rotates 360 degrees around the area to be scanned. Each CT slice is obtained independently from the others, and each slice can be rescanned if movement occurs to blur the X-ray (Filipek et al., 1992). The time required for a scan is approximately 15 to 20 minutes. The advantages of CT scans are the relatively short time it takes to scan the person, the lower cost, and the ability to repeat individual slices. The disadvantages of CT scans are that the temporal lobes are not readily scanned using this technique, the clarity of the picture and structures is inferior to that of the MRI, and radiation is necessary to produce the images (Filipek & Blickman, 1992).

MRI allows the visualization of the brain at about the clarity level of an autopsy. An MRI is a large magnet with a strong magnetic field. The patient lies on a movable table, which goes inside a doughnut-hole-like opening. A headpiece covers the brain to be scanned, allowing an opening over the face. The physics underlying MRI involve the alignment of hydrogen photons in the same direction as the magnetic field. A radio frequency pulse deflects the photons to an angle predetermined by the clinician. Once the pulse ceases, the photons return to their original alignment through a series of ever-relaxing circles (Filipek & Blickman, 1992). By altering the rate, duration, and intensity of the radio frequency pulses, the visualization of the brain can be changed. There are several sequences that an MRI scan requires, each of which averages 7 to 10 minutes in length.

MRI utilizes T_1- and T_2-weighted scans. T_1-weighted scans provide excellent visualization of myelin and structures, with white matter showing as white and gray matter as gray. T_2-weighted scans are more sensitive to water content in the tissues and more readily able to visualize the extent of lesions, with white matter showing darker than gray matter. MRI does not use radiation and is fairly risk-free; however, it is expensive and is generally used only when a CT scan is inconclusive or there is a suspicion of a brain abnormality not picked up by the CT scan. Before the advent of this technology, neuropsychological assessment was utilized to localize tumors, lesions, and the like. MRI scans are now used for this process, and neuropsychological assessment is used for intervention planning and in determining how the person solves problems (Semrud-Clikeman & Griffin, 2000).

MRI scans are not able to pinpoint damage at the microcellular level. For example, a follow-up study of children with moderate or severe TBI found neuropsychological deficits in the absence of MRI-discovered pathology (Levin et al., 1993). Such findings were suggested to be related to decreased cerebral blood flow rather than structural abnormalities (Newton et al., 1992).

Functional MRI (fMRI) is an emerging clinical technique that is currently used mostly for research. It allows for the mapping of cerebral blood flow, as well as changes in this flow and oxygenation (Posner & Raichle, 1994). It allows for the study of brain activation through a technique that provides an image of the blood flow. Contrast agents are utilized to visualize these systems and are fairly risk-free. This technique shows promise for evaluating children who continue to show neuropsychological deficits in the face of normal MRI/CT findings.

A neurological examination generally involves an in-depth review of the patient's medical and developmental history, an assessment of mental status, an assessment of the cranial nerves and motor and sensory systems, and an assessment of the autonomic nervous system (Swaiman, 1994a). Muscle tone, coordination, and reflexes are also assessed. During the presentation of the developmental history, the child is generally present and the neurologist notes the child's attention, language, and affect, as well as parent–child interactions. Swaiman (1994a) suggests that the physician ask him/herself the following questions: Does the child respond positively to the parent's interactions? Does the child attempt to manipulate the parent? Is the response transient or persistent? Is the parent's attitude one of caring or hostility? Reflexes are checked to determine spinal and cerebellar functioning. Motor coordination is also checked by having the child walk a straight line, balance on one foot, run smoothly, and hop. Sensory systems are checked by the doctor's touching the child, who has his/her eyes closed, in various places with either a finger or a tuning fork. The child is also asked to recognize various objects that are placed in his/her hand with eyes closed. Difficulty in performing these tasks implicates the parietal lobe but can also indicate problems with attention. Muscle strength is also assessed by having the child push against the neurologist's hand and stand without additional help. Positive signs (abnormality) found during this evaluation generally result in a referral for an MRI or CT scan.

To more fully understand the mechanisms underlying TBI, it is important to briefly review neuroanatomy. The purpose of this book is not to provide an extensive review of physiological psychology, which many of you had in your master's or doctoral programs. Rather, the following chapter is intended to refresh your memory in this area before the neuropsychological and educational needs of children with TBI are discussed.

CHAPTER 2

◆◆◆

Functional Neuroanatomy

◆

Children with TBI experience damage in either a focal or a diffuse manner. Focal injury involves a specified area of the brain; diffuse injury involves several areas or networks. A focal injury can also implicate adjacent areas, depending on the site and the force of the injury. In children, the brain is continuing to develop, and thus a developmental approach is important for our understanding. There is a developmental difference between injury experienced at age 1 and at age 10, particularly in outcome. The following sections provide a brief summary of neuroanatomy from a functional standpoint, including the various areas of the brain and the main functions of these areas.

CENTRAL NERVOUS SYSTEM

The nervous system is divided into two basic systems: the central nervous system (CNS) and the peripheral nervous system (PNS). The CNS is made up of the brain and the spinal cord and is completely encased in bone. The PNS connects the CNS to the rest of the body through spinal, cranial, and peripheral nerves. Although the PNS is an important system of the brain, we are mainly concerned with the CNS and, particularly, the brain.

The CNS is surrounded by cerebrospinal fluid (CSF) to cushion the brain against trauma and to provide a barrier, called the blood–brain barrier, against unwanted chemicals traveling through the bloodstream. CSF, a colorless solution of sodium chloride and other salts, is produced in the ventricles, which are interconnected spaces in the brain. There are two lateral ventricles in the cerebrum, a third ventricle in the juncture between the cerebrum and the brainstem, and the fourth ventricle in the brainstem. The ventricles enlarge as a function of some diseases (e.g., encephalitis, meningi-

16

tis) or head injury, and such enlargement can cause additional damage (Levin et al., 1995).

CSF is present within the meninges, which form the lining of the brain and spinal cord and serve as protection. The meninges are of three types: pia mater, subarachnoid space, and dura mater. The dura mater ("tough mother") is the outer covering of the brain. The subarachnoid space is between the dura and pia and is filled with CSF. The pia mater ("soft mother") is the innermost lining of the brain and spinal cord.

The brain is composed of approximately 180 billion cells, 50 billion of which are responsible for transmitting and receiving sensory–motor signals (Kolb & Whishaw, 1990). There are two major types of cells in the CNS, the neurons and the neuroglia. Neurons are the conductors of nerve impulses; the neuroglia provide the structural support and insulation of the synapses between cells and produce the cerebrospinal fluid that cushions the brain and spinal cord from the jars and jolts of everyday living.

Neurons are made up of axons, dendrites, cell bodies, and axon terminals (see Figure 2.1). The cell bodies, the neuroglia, and the blood vessels of the CNS are gray in color and constitute the gray matter of the brain. Myelin, which covers the long axons, is known as the white matter of the

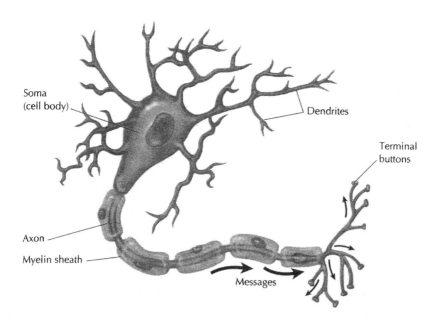

FIGURE 2.1. Structures of a neuron. From Neil R. Carlson, *Physiology of Behavior* (5th ed.). Copyright 1994 by Allyn & Bacon. Reprinted by permission.

brain. The cell body contains the ribonucleic acid (RNA) and deoxyribonucleic acid (DNA) of the cell and is the life center of a neuron. RNA is responsible for protein synthesis in the cell and transmits instructions about necessary metabolic functions. DNA contains the genetic blueprint for the cell. The cell body also includes a nucleus and ribosomes. The nucleus of the cell includes the chromosomes and the nucleolus, which manufactures ribosomes that are involved in protein synthesis. The bulk of the cell is cytoplasm, made up of many cells, which is a dynamic structure containing the mitochondria. The mitochondria are shaped like beads and are responsible for the energy production for the cell. Destruction of the cell body can cause the death of the neuron.

The dendrites branch off the cell bodies and receive impulses from other neurons (Rayport, 1992). The dendrites continue to grow during childhood, forming dendritic spines and synapses to communicate with other cells. Failure to form dendritic spines has been implicated in mental retardation (Kandel et al., 1993). The axons are covered with myelin, a fatty substance that allows for the rapid transmission of impulses. Axons carry the messages away from the cell body and toward another cell body. Although most axons are myelinated at the time of birth, myelination continues throughout childhood. Changes in brain weight up to the age of 8 to 10 years are related to increases in dendritic connections and myelin (Shepard, 1994).

The axons end in terminal branches that form a synapse (see Figure 2.1). A synapse allows nerve impulses to move from one nerve to another through the release of chemicals referred to as *neurotransmitters*. Thousands of synapses are present, and each dendritic spine serves as a synapse for other axons. When a neuron receives a message from another neuron, neurotransmitters are released and influence the activity of the receiving cell. Extra neurotransmitters are either reabsorbed by the synapse or recycled through the CSF.

The brain is divided into three major divisions: the brainstem, the cerebellum, and the cortex. Each of these divisions has specific functions, and damage to any of these areas can result in specific deficits. The limbic system and basal ganglia are also part of the CNS. Figure 2.2 provides an illustration of the major brain structures.

Brainstem

The brainstem consists of five areas: fourth ventricle, medulla oblongata, pons, midbrain, and diencephalon. The *fourth ventricle*, also referred to as the aqueduct of Sylvius, is filled with cerebrospinal fluid (Brodal, 1992). Enlargement of the ventricle can signal the presence of a disease process such as encephalitis or meningitis, as well as increased intracerebral pressure.

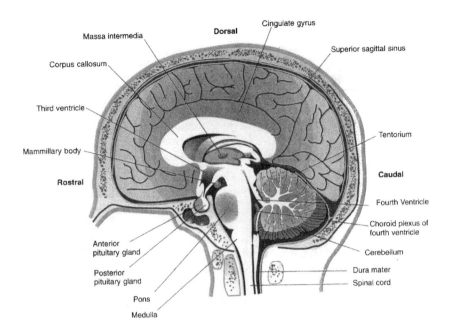

FIGURE 2.2. Midsagittal view of the brain and pertinent structures. From Neil R. Carlson, *Physiology of Behavior* (5th ed.). Copyright 1994 by Allyn & Bacon. Reprinted by permission.

The *medulla oblongata* sits above the spinal cord and contains groups of sensory and motor nuclei and several of the cranial nerves. Sensory and motor tracts cross in the medulla. The reticular activating system (RAS) is also present in the medulla and is responsible for control of blood pressure, blood volume in organs, and heart rate, as well as wakefulness and regulation of sleep (Brodal, 1992). The RAS is richly connected to all levels of the CNS and modulates its activity through maintaining consciousness and attentional states in the brain (Reitan & Wolfson, 1985b; Sagvolden & Archer, 1989). Anesthetics appear to work on the RAS. In addition, the RAS projects to the portion of the limbic system that serves the behavioral and emotional mechanisms of pain.

The *pons* is between the medulla and the midbrain and serves as a bridge across the right and left hemispheres. Major sensory and motor pathways course through the pons and enter the higher cortical regions. The pons, in coordination with the cerebellum, receives information from the motor cortex and assists in modulating movement. In addition, input from the limbic system to the pons has been thought to affect motivation to begin an action. The secretion of serotonin, an important neurotransmitter, as well as norepinephrine, a modulator for other neurotransmitters takes place in the pons (Comings, 1990). The continuation of the RAS in the pons appears to be important in sleep modulation.

The *diencephalon* of the brain is responsible for the integration of sensory experiences and relaying the resulting responses (Kolb & Whishaw, 1990). It includes the thalamus, the hypothalamus, the pituitary gland, the internal capsule, the third ventricle, and the optic nerve (Brodal, 1992) (see Figure 2.2). The thalamus is responsible for relaying visual, auditory, motor, and sensory information to the cerebrum; it is a way station for nerve impulses and radiates into the frontal, temporal, and occipital cortices. The hypothalamus plays a role in modulating and controlling emotions, sexual functions, eating, temperature, and thirst, as well as contributing to rage and violence reactions. The pituitary is governed by the hypothalamus and releases hormones regulating bodily functions. The internal capsule contains the fibers connecting the cortex to the brainstem and spinal cord, and the frontal lobe to the thalamus and pons.

Cerebellum

The cerebellum connects to the midbrain, pons, and medulla. It receives sensory information about the position of limbs in space as well as input as to muscle alignment. This structure is important for coordinated, smooth, and complex motor activity. Injury to the cerebellum can result in movement disorders, slurred speech, blurred vision and dizziness, and loss of muscle tone (Swaiman, 1994b). Tumors involving the cerebellum and fourth ventricle, although rare, are the most frequent type of tumor in childhood (Cohen & Duffner, 2000).

Limbic System

The limbic system is a deep structure in the cerebrum; it includes the hippocampus, amygdala, and cingulate gyrus. It has widespread connections to all areas of the cortex and to the endocrine system. It appears to serve as a relay area for cognitive and emotional input (Wilkinson, 1986). The limbic system also appears to coordinate reactions to pleasant, frightening, or threatening experiences, to monitor sexual response, and to store information in long-term memory. The hippocampus is located near the temporal lobe, an area particularly vulnerable to damage from traumatic head injury. Damage to the hippocampus has been implicated in the inability to store new memories or to learn new things. Feelings of fear and violent behavior have been associated with damage to the amygdala. Aggression and indifference to social mores, as well as obsessive–compulsive symptoms, have been associated with lesions to the cingulate gyrus. Seizure activity in the limbic structures sometimes spreads to temporal lobe structures, resulting in a temporary loss of consciousness and memory (Lockman, 1994).

Basal Ganglia

The basal ganglia are the masses of gray matter that are enclosed in the cerebral hemispheres and generally surrounded by white matter. They include the caudate nucleus, putamen, and globus pallidus (Shepard, 1994). The basal ganglia serve to connect the cortex with the thalamus, the midbrain structures, and the spinal cord. This area is also intimately connected to the prefrontal region and the limbic system (Comings, 1990). These serotonin-rich pathways inhibit motor actions and emotional responses. The caudate has been implicated in ADHD through MRI studies (Filipek et al., 1998; Semrud-Clikeman et al., 2000). Damage to this area produces postural changes, hypo or hyper muscle tone, and movement disorders such as tremors or jerks (Ashwal & Schneider, 1994).

Cortex

The cortex contains the most highly developed system and constitutes approximately 80% of the human brain (Kolb & Whishaw, 1990). The cortex consists of ridges (gyri) and valleys (sulci); the deepest indentations are called *fissures*. The lateral (or Sylvian) fissure separates the frontal lobe from the temporal lobe, and the central sulcus separates the frontal from the parietal lobe (see Figure 2.2). The central sulcus separates the motor from the sensory cortex and is a major landmark. The cortex is composed of right and left hemispheres, which have anatomical as well as functional differences (Brodal, 1992; Semrud-Clikeman & Hynd, 1991). *Lateralization* refers to the extent that each hemisphere is specialized for certain types of tasks. The left hemisphere has more gray matter than white matter, as compared with the right hemisphere, which has the converse proportion.

The left hemisphere has more short association fibers, which allow for the processing of serial or sequential material more readily, as used in language and reading tasks (Teeter & Semrud-Clikeman, 1997). The right hemisphere has longer connections and appears to process more readily those materials that require wholistic analysis (Goldberg & Costa, 1981). Thus, social understanding and processing of novel information appear to be typically right hemisphere tasks. It is currently hypothesized that the two hemispheres can operate independently of each other in some domain-specific functions, whereas interaction between the hemispheres is present at particular stages of processing, thus allowing for flexibility and adaptability (Zaidel et al., 1990).

Damage to the left hemisphere can result in a shift of language functions to the right hemisphere following TBI, particularly if damage is present in both the frontal and temporal lobes (Kolb & Fantie, 1989). Although language functions can be absorbed by the right hemisphere, complex visual–spatial functions (usually right hemispheric functions) are compromised, as well as complex syntactic processing (Scheibel, 1990). Thus, although there is some ability of the hemispheres to switch functions, the cost is a compromise of higher-level functions.

The cortex is composed of four lobes in each hemisphere: frontal, parietal, occipital, and temporal. The frontal lobe includes the motor cortex, the parietal the somatosensory cortex, the temporal (auditory) cortex, and the occipital (visual) cortex. Figure 2.3 presents these lobes.

Frontal Lobes

The frontal lobes are the most anterior region and include the primary motor cortex, the premotor cortex, the center for oral speech (Broca's area), and the prefrontal cortex. The primary motor cortex allows for the execu-

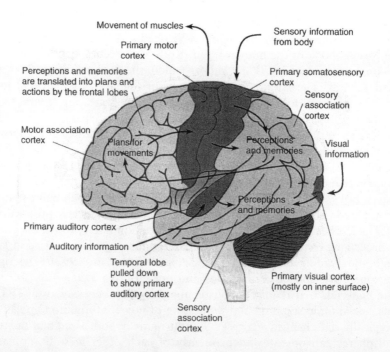

FIGURE 2.3. View of the lobes and the connections between the sensory and motor cortices. From Neil R. Carlson, *Physiology of Behavior* (5th ed.). Copyright 1994 by Allyn & Bacon. Reprinted by permission.

tion of simple motor functions, including fine motor and highly skilled voluntary movements (Ghez, 1993). It receives input from the parietal lobe, cerebellum, and thalamus for the integration of sensory and motor input. Specific muscle groups are represented along the central sulcus, and stimulation to these areas produces muscle contracture (Kolb & Whishaw, 1990). Injury to the motor cortex can result in paralysis of the opposite side of the body.

The premotor cortex is anterior to the motor cortex and controls limb and body movements. Attentional and motivation aspects of motor movement are also controlled in this area in conjunction with the limbic system. The premotor cortex is responsible for directing the primary motor cortex in more complex and integrated movements. Premotor cortex damage results in coordination problems in complex motor actions. Children and adults with impairment in this region generally experience difficulty imitating two-part movements (patting the head with one hand while rubbing the stomach with the other hand). In addition, there may be difficulty in pronouncing multisyllabic words, even while the ability to pronounce individual speech sounds is spared. Moreover, deficits in this region lead to perseveration in writing (i.e., writing the same sentence or word over and over again). In addition, the frontal cortex includes the region for oral speech, also called Broca's area.

The prefrontal cortex is the most anterior region of the frontal lobe. It is richly connected to the limbic system, as well as to the thalamus and hypothalamus. The control and regulation of affect is a primary function of the prefrontal cortex. In addition, connections to the association regions of the brain (where the occipital, temporal, and parietal lobes converge) provide the ability to compare and contrast present and past experiences. The ability to use insight and judgment to guide one's behavior is also a function of the prefrontal region. These abilities, often referred to as executive functions, include planning, organization, and evaluation of one's own behavior. Impairment in the prefrontal regions often results in poor inhibition, impaired executive functions and judgment, and, at times, intellectual deficits (Tranel, 1992). Increased apathy, lowered activity level, and perseveration can also be observed. Moreover, commands—even though repeated by the individual—do not direct behavior. There is an accompanying lack of insight into problems as well as difficulty in organization and planning. Interpersonal problems are often present, as the person may become unduly critical of others but have little insight into his/her own behavior.

Parietal Lobes

The parietal lobes are demarcated by the central sulcus and the Sylvian fissure. The main role of the parietal lobes is the perception of tactile information in the form of pain recognition, pressure and touch sensation, and knowledge of where a limb is in space. There are three functional areas to the parietal lobes: primary, secondary, and association. The primary sensory cortex is immediately posterior to the central sulcus. This area has been found to be highly interrelated with the closely lying motor cortex (Woolsey, 1958).

The primary sensory cortex is responsible for the recognition of pain, discrimination of vibration and touch, and the awareness of body position. Similar to the primary motor cortex, the primary sensory cortex is also arranged by body region, with areas requiring more sensory input (tongue, lips, mouth) being distributed in a larger area. Injury to this region produces sensory deficits, in the particular region damaged, in the opposite side of the body.

The secondary parietal area integrates more complex sensory information from the primary parietal area. The association area is involved in complex sensory information and synthesizes information received from the primary and secondary areas. This area overlaps with the association areas of the temporal and occipital lobes. Although damage to this area does not result in sensory deficits, it does affect the ability to integrate complex sensory information. The ability to pair visual and auditory stimuli with sensory information is harmed. Thus, the ability to identify objects by touch is impaired. Damage to the parietal lobes is generally not readily apparent. There are differences in right and left parietal lobe functions. Damage to the association area of the right hemisphere results in difficulty in identifying objects by feel and with figure copying. People with deficits in this area also frequently experience difficulty with directionality and may easily get lost and confused about space. Damage to the association area of the left hemisphere results in difficulty in following directions involving more than one step, difficulty with speech and syntax, problems with left–right discrimination, problems in imitating body actions, and some difficulty in motor planning.

Occipital Lobes

The occipital lobes form the most posterior portion of the cortex. Like the parietal lobes, the occipital lobes are divided into primary, secondary, and association areas. The primary occipital cortex receives information from the thalamus through pathways that transverse the temporal lobe. These pathways are responsible for visual input to the cortex, and damage to this pathway at any point produces defects in the visual field. The secondary region allows for finer visual discrimination. Deficits in this area result in difficulty in recognizing objects by sight, inability to attend to more than one aspect of a visual stimulus at a time, and difficulty in recognizing colors. The association area allows for complex visual perception, as well as integration of other sensory information. Damage in this region in the right hemisphere can produce visual deficits that include an inability to recognize faces, objects, or drawings. Difficulty in the left occipital association area can result in problems in recognizing a complex pattern, drawing a complex figure as a whole, and reversing numbers and letters; and in the right occipital association area, problems with understanding ownership.

Temporal Lobes

The temporal lobes also have three divisions: primary, secondary, and association. The temporal lobes have many connections to the other lobes through several major pathways. One pathway is particularly important; it connects the temporal and frontal lobes (arcuate fasciculus) and is necessary for the pairing of expressive and receptive language. The temporal lobes are responsible for the perception of auditory information, analysis of the affective tone of a communication, and long-term memory storage. The temporal lobe of the left hemisphere is important in understanding language, and that of the right hemisphere is implicated in understanding the intent of a speaker as well as recognizing faces and gestures (Semrud-Clikeman & Hynd, 1990).

The function of the primary temporal cortex is to perceive speech sounds (in the left hemisphere) and tone patterns (in the right hemisphere). The ability to make sound–symbol relationships is a function of the secondary temporal cortex. The secondary temporal cortex is also involved in auditory discrimination of finer sounds. The association area is involved in the ability to pair these discriminations with parietal and occipital information and is implicated in the reading process, thought to be localized at the angular gyrus. Damage to this region can cause difficulty with receptive language, poor reading comprehension, and poor ability to repeat information.

In addition to auditory processing, the temporal cortex is also involved in memory processes in conjunction with the hippocampus and amygdala. These areas have been linked to the ability to learn new material and to lay down new memories (Tranel, 1992). The ability to recall verbal information presented either visually or orally is a left-hemispheric function, and the ability to recall nonverbal information (geometric drawings, faces, etc.) is a right hemispheric function. Damage to the temporal/hippocampal region results in an inability to learn new material, as new memories are unable to be stored (Kupfermann, 1991).

Conclusion

Knowledge of the functional neuroanatomy of the brain is important for an understanding of what occurs in TBI. It is particularly relevant for school and clinical practitioners in understanding the reports of medical personnel using such terms as *white matter, frontal lobes, central sulcus,* and so on, to describe the damage experienced by a child. Practitioners must also pay attention to the developing brain in pediatric TBI, which differs from adult brain injury in that respect. A developmental approach is crucial to our understanding of the damage that has been done, as well as the possible outcomes. Moreover, as discussed in the following chapters, damage to a particular area of the brain does not result in the same symptoms for all individuals. Brains are like fingerprints, in that each is unique, and the outcome of disruption to a certain set of neurons will differ between individuals. Therefore, it is important to understand and recognize patterns usually associated with specific regions, but also to maintain a openness to symptoms that may not be consistent with damage to a particular site.

DEVELOPMENT OF THE BRAIN

There is an orderliness in the development of the brain, with mechanisms most necessary to survival developing first. The primary motor system of the brain is the first to develop and is operational at birth (Hynd & Willis, 1988). This system allows the child to suck on a bottle or breast and obtain nourishment. As explained earlier, the primary motor system is in the frontal lobe. Just posterior to the motor system is the sensory system, which is believed to develop concurrently with the motor unit (Martin, 1993). Rapid maturation of the brain in this area, particularly in the right hemisphere, has been found from 1 month of age to age 2 or 3 (Hashimoto et al., 1995). Development of the primary visual system, which is slower in humans than in other primates, is next (Hynd & Willis, 1988). The neurons in this system are fairly well myelinated by 6 weeks of age and are fully developed by 3 months (Kolb & Fantie, 1989). The primary auditory system develops between the ages of 1 and 4 months to allow infants to begin to differentiate between speech sounds (Eimas, 1985). Functional lateralization of the left hemisphere in infants has been found for speech sounds and in the right hemisphere for music and nonspeech sounds (Molfese & Molfese, 1986).

Growth spurts in the lobes occur throughout the preschool years, with increases in cortical connections between the lobes seen at three time periods: (1) age 1.5–5 years; (2) 5–10 years; (3) 10–14 years (Thatcher, 1991,

1994). In the left hemisphere there is a lengthening of connections between the posterior association regions and the frontal lobe, and in the right hemisphere the long myelinated fibers shorten with development. Thatcher (1994) suggests that the left hemisphere is expanding to accommodate new functional systems while the right hemisphere is consolidating existing systems.

Language areas also exhibit a developmental gradient. The right motor speech area initially shows greater dendritic growth. As you may recall, the infant uses affective nonverbal speech to communicate (crying, fussing, smiling). As language develops, the dendritic growth shifts to the left hemisphere and increases dramatically over the first 3 years of life. The temporal lobes also increase in myelination at this time, and this increase is particularly evident in the auditory association areas and in the region responsible for sound–symbol association (Hynd & Willis, 1988).

Tactile perception increases over the course of development. Preschool children are beginning to develop hand preference, and improvement in tactile perception occurs between the ages of 8 and 12, particularly for the preferred hand. Prior to age 9, children experience difficulty in correctly identifying a touch on a specific finger, and most preschool children are unable to complete this task (Benton et al., 1983). By the age of 9 most children can identify a finger that is touched. When verbal responses are required to identify a touch to the right hand, accuracy is increased. Conversely, nonverbal responses increase accuracy with the left hand (Bakker, 1972).

Visual recognition of complex figures also develops throughout the preschool period. Facial recognition has been found to be a right hemispheric task in children as young as 4 years (Kolb & Fantie, 1989). Matching facial expressions to situations is a more associative task and is not well developed until the age of 14 (Kolb & Fantie, 1989).

More complex functions require a longer period for development, and many of them require development of the frontal lobes. The frontal lobes are believed to continue to develop up to age 49 (Teeter & Semrud-Clikeman, 1997). The frontal lobes are believed to involve complex cognitive functions, including regulation of affect, planning and organization, and insight into a person's own behavior (sometimes referred to as executive functions).

A THEORETICAL FRAMEWORK FOR DEVELOPMENT

Luria (1980) provides a theoretical framework to assist in our understanding of the development of higher cortical functions. Based on his research, Luria proposes three units of the brain that develop both simultaneously and sequentially: the arousal unit, the sensory-input unit, and the organizational and planning unit (Willis & Widerstrom, 1986).

Unit I: Arousal Unit

The arousal unit has many neural connections to the frontal lobe; it is made up of the brainstem and contains the RAS. This unit is specialized to provide cortical tone and arousal through the RAS. When cortical tone is too low, the brain becomes unable to distinguish between various stimuli or, in other cases, to filter out extraneous information. The RAS prevents the brain from being flooded by irrelevant information while providing optimum arousal for information processing. If the RAS should filter out too much information, sensory deprivation can occur, requiring the cortex to generate its own stimulation (Teeter & Semrud-Clikeman, 1997). Substantial damage at this level can interfere with consciousness. Less severe damage can result in disorganization, distractibility, attentional deficits, and insomnia. Unit I is believed to develop during the first year of life and continue to exert influence until adolescence, when higher-order units take over.

Unit II: Sensory-Input Unit

Unit II is composed of the temporal, occipital, and parietal lobes. The major function of this region is sensory reception and integration and corresponds to the sensory modality of the lobe (parietal—somatosensory; occipital—visual; temporal—auditory). Luria hypothesizes that Unit II is guided by three functional laws: (1) Change is present in these regions throughout development; (2) these regions decrease in specificity with development; and (3) lateralization increases during development (Luria, 1980).

The lobes are each divided into three zones: primary, secondary, and tertiary. The primary zones sort and record information. The secondary zones organize the sensory information and store it for later retrieval. The tertiary zones integrate the data from various sources and lay the basis for organized behavior. Intelligence tests are hypothesized to measure mostly Unit II tasks. The function of Unit II to code, analyze, and store information corresponds well to the verbal portion of intelligence tests. For more novel tasks, such as those contained in the performance subtests of the third edition of the Wechsler Intelligence Scale for Children (WISC-III; Wechsler, 1991), higher-level functions may be necessary.

Primary Zones

Primary zones involve sense receptors and have relationships to the appropriate sensory organs. These zones are hardwired at birth and determined by genetics. In the temporal lobe the primary zone involves the auditory modality; in the occipital, vision; in the frontal, the motor function; and in the parietal lobe, the somatosensory modality.

Secondary Zones

The secondary zones in each of the three lobes are involved in reception and integration of the sensory data. It is believed that these zones process information sequentially. In the temporal lobe, the secondary zone is involved in the analysis and synthesis of sounds and the analysis of intonation, pitch, and rhythm. The parietal lobe secondary zone is involved in two-point discrimination, movement detection, and the recognition of objects by feel. Finally, the occipital lobe secondary zone is involved in visual discrimination of letters, shapes, and figures. The secondary areas begin development at birth and continue through adolescence. Unit II is most dominant in development during the elementary and middle school years as knowledge is laid down for further use.

Consistent with Luria's hypotheses, lateralization occurs more extensively in the secondary zones as development occurs. In the left hemisphere, the secondary zones are responsible for analyzing verbal information and in the right hemisphere are responsible for music, environmental sounds, and language prosody. Reading is a bihemispheric task, with the right hemisphere involved in the initial learning of letters and words and the left hemisphere mostly responsible for the act of reading once the basic skills have become automatized. In addition, the left hemisphere processes the sequential aspects of language and the right hemisphere is responsible for analyzing the emotional tone of that language (Teeter & Semrud-Clikeman, 1997). Writing also becomes lateralized, with the right hemisphere activated when a novel visual–motor task is presented, and the left hemisphere engaged once the task has been learned.

Tertiary Zones

The tertiary zones allow for cross-modal integration of information from all sensory modalities. The tertiary zones are generally believed to process information simultaneously. Intelligence tests tap the tertiary areas most heavily, and damage to this region can result in problems with learning, lower intelligence, and poorer understanding of language. The tertiary zones generally mature from the age of 5 to early adulthood (Golden, 1981).

Unit III: Organizational and Planning Unit

Unit III is composed of the frontal lobes and can be also divided into three zones. Thus unit requires the longest developmental span and is generally believed to begin developing in early adolescence through early adulthood. Some authors suggest that Unit III continues to develop into a person's 30s or 40s (Golden, 1981; Hynd & Willis, 1988). This unit is specialized for goal-directed behavior as well planning and organization. The primary zone of Unit III involves the motor strip and is involved in simple motor output. The secondary zone of Unit III is the premotor region and is involved in motor and speech sequencing. The third zone is localized to the orbitofrontal region and is the last area to myelinate and develop.

The tertiary zone is involved with planning, organization, and evaluation of behavior (executive functions). Damage to this region is believed to be related to problems in delaying gratification, poor impulse control, difficulty in learning from past mistakes, and attentional deficits (Lezak, 1994; Teeter & Semrud-Clikeman, 1997). In addition, development of Unit III can compensate for deficits in Unit I. This compensation may involve the ability to control behavior such as overactivity through conscious thought. For example, historically it was believed that children outgrew ADHD by age 15 or 16. We now know that ADHD generally continues, but that the presentation may change with age (Barkley, 1998). For some children and adolescents, medication can be reduced or eliminated at older ages—this is not due to "recovery" from ADHD, but rather to the ability of Unit III to direct behavior in a purposeful manner (Teeter, 1998).

Conclusion

The brain is designed to develop throughout life, with special networks laid down for integration of the information gathered throughout a person's life span. These networks become increasingly proficient with age and with use and require fewer connections to work with efficiency. When normal development is interrupted either through a head injury, a genetic process, or an environmental insult, the brain compensates in many ways. However, even with such compensation, the efficiency of the CNS can be compromised. The areas that are particularly vulnerable to damage are the orbitofrontal region of the frontal lobes (the area at the front of the skull) and the temporal poles of the temporal lobe. Brain functions that are susceptible to damage include attention, planning and organization, executive functions, and memory, as well as social, behavioral, and emotional adjustment. These abilities are discussed in the following chapter.

CHAPTER 3

◆◆◆

Neuropsychological Correlates

◆

As the child develops, more complex intellectual abilities are expected. The consolidation of early learning into propositional networks allows for the efficient storage and retrieval of previously learned material (Woolfolk, 2001). Such consolidation requires the ability to pay attention to a task, to code information, and to retrieve information in a timely manner. At any of these points, disruption in the neural basis for learning can negatively affect the ability to lay down new networks or retrieve information already learned. As discussed in Chapter 1, the age of the child and the severity and region of damage all determine the intellectual functions that are disrupted. In addition, some intellectual functions, such as advanced executive functioning, are not expected at an early age, and deficits in these areas may not appear until later in life. Kolb and Fantie (1989) suggest that damage to the frontal and posterior brain regions may not be identified until the child is more than 12 to 15 years of age. In other cases early damage to the temporal lobe or to association areas involved in the reading process may not be evident until the child begins to learn how to read. In addition, younger children may show difficulty with attention, impulsivity, and lability rather than cognitive deficits following an injury, whereas older children show the opposite pattern (Rourke et al., 1983). It has been suggested that early attention problems may mask the cognitive deficits seen at a later time when certain developmental stages are appropriate and expected (Rourke et al., 1983).

Deficits resulting from damage that occurs in late childhood or adolescence generally resemble deficits seen in adults (Teeter & Semrud-Clikeman, 1997). Areas that are most frequently compromised in TBI include intelligence, perception, memory, attention, and psychosocial functioning (Ewing-Cobbs et al., 1986). In some children, the damage is lateralized and one or two of these areas are involved. In more severely involved children, many of these areas can be affected and the prognosis is far more guarded.

Dikeman and colleagues (1986) evaluated 45 adolescent and adult patients with mild to moderate head injuries, using a standard neuropsychological battery (the Halstead–Reitan). These authors concluded that more complex cognitive functions appear to be affected more severely than lower-level skills (e.g., reading comprehension vs. word recognition). These skills can also include social judgment, planning, organization, and the ability to learn from past mistakes. Dikeman and colleagues also found that improvement occurs in both complex and simple cognitive tasks, and for children and adolescents improvement can be seen for up to 5 years after injury—for adults maximum recovery is generally seen within the first 18 months following the injury (Lezak, 1994).

INTELLECTUAL FUNCTIONING

Intellectual deficits following TBI are more common in children with severe brain injury and who were in a coma for more than 24 hours (Fletcher et al., 1995). In addition, a child's age at the time of injury also plays a role in intellectual development. In the past it was believed that injury to the younger brain did not have serious cognitive ramifications. However, more recent work indicates that early brain injury may be related to long-term cognitive deficits, particularly if the damage is multifocal and diffuse (Dennis & Barnes, 1990). It has been suggested that the previous belief that there were few cognitive deficits with early brain injury has frequently forestalled the cognitive evaluation of young children with TBI, perhaps causing an underestimate of the degree to which such deficits exist (Dennis et al., 1995). Similarly, age has been found to be an important variable for the treatment of leukemia and of brain tumors, with younger children showing more cognitive deficits following radiation than those who are older (Dennis et al., 1995; Semrud-Clikeman, 1999).

The amount of time since the occurrence of damage is another important variable. The relationship between damage and intelligence has been found to change over time, with decreasing IQ scores found in children with focal lesions (Banich et al., 1990). Children experiencing brain injury before age 3 have shown lower IQ scores than those experiencing damage in late childhood and adolescence (Aram & Eisele, 1994; Nass et al., 1989). Dennis and colleagues (1995) suggest that these findings indicate that a lower IQ may be indicative of difficulty in consolidating information into a complex knowledge base. These authors further recommend that children with head injuries be serially evaluated to document possible cognitive changes over time.

Studies have found that the performance IQ (PIQ) of the Wechsler Intelligence Scale for Children (WISC) is particularly vulnerable to TBI (Dalby & Obrzut, 1991). Begali (1992) indicates that the deficits initially seen on the PIQ of the WISC continue, although not at the same magnitude as measured directly following the injury, whereas the verbal IQ (VIQ) shows improvement at the premorbid level. These findings are consistent with those of Chadwick and colleagues (1981b), who found a 10-point drop in VIQ immediately following a head injury and a *30-point* drop in PIQ. The VIQ was found to be at premorbid levels 1 year postinjury, whereas a 10-point decrease continued to be found in PIQ.

The ability to solve new problems is one of the areas of intellectual deficit identified by several researchers to be more susceptible to damage than acquired knowledge (Chadwick et al., 1981b; Levin & Eisenberg, 1979; Winogron et al., 1984). Further support for the relationship between lowered IQ and brain injury comes from a quantitative MRI study of two groups with moderate to severe closed-head injury (Bigler et al., 1999). This study found structural differences in the patients with lower IQs (full scale IQ, FSIQ, less than 90) including enlarged ventricles and temporal/subcortical atrophy. Those with higher IQs did not show compromised structures.

Donders and Warschausky (1996, 1997) evaluated the use of four factors of the WISC-III (Wechsler, 1991) in assessing children with TBI. For their sample, the verbal comprehension (VC) and freedom from distractibility (FD) factors were present. However, these factors were not found to be related to severity of head injury (Donders, 1995). Lower scores on the processing speed (PS) and perceptual organization (PO) factors were related to severity of TBI. To determine whether the difficulty present on the PIQ was due to visual–spatial deficits or speed-of-performance difficulties was not clear.

Donders (1997) studied children with mild, moderate, and severe head injuries. The severe group was found to have statistically lower scores on the PIQ, PS, and PO measures as compared with the other two groups. The mild and moderate groups did not differ from each other on any of the measures. Moreover, selective impairment on the PO and PS indices was found to be specific to the TBI group but not to the WISC-III standardization sample (Donders, 1996; Donders & Warschausky, 1996; Hoffman et al., 2000).

There were differences in the patterns of factors in the Donders and Warshausky (1996) study. The most distinct pattern was found for a group of children scoring poorly on the PO and PS indices, as compared with low average scores on the VC and FD factors. These children were found to be disproportionately in the severe head injury group and showed diffuse lesions on CT/MRI scans, with the predominance of the lesions present in the right hemisphere. This finding was interpreted to mean that damage to the right hemisphere, particularly to the white matter, in these children resulted in poorer visual–spatial and fluid reasoning skills.

These findings argue for a sensitivity to a intellectual profile that is specific to TBI and that the consistent finding of PIQ differences is an important factor that should be carefully evaluated by school personnel. Difficulty in processing information quickly and in solving novel problems may certainly affect functioning in later elementary and high school grades. These findings have implications for school reentry as well as outcome.

ACADEMIC FUNCTIONING

It has been fairly well documented that children with TBI show difficulties with language and reading, arithmetic calculation, writing, and spelling (Levin, Ewing-Cobbs, & Eisenberg, 1995). According to the National Institutes on Health (NIH, 1998), these difficulties frequently go unrecognized in both the adult and pediatric populations. The NIH Consensus Development Panel on Rehabilitation of Persons with Traumatic Brain Injury (1998) also states that the needs of children with TBI may not fit into the "typical school educational programs" (p. 4), as many such children exhibit a need for special education. The effectiveness of programs for children with TBI was reported to be poorly studied, as was our ability to adequately evaluate their needs.

A longitudinal study of children with TBI aged 5 to 11 years found that those with severe TBI achieved poorer reading recognition, spelling, and arithmetic scores than those with mild to moderate TBI (Ewing-Cobbs et al., 1998a). The older children were found to score lower on measures of numerical operations and reading comprehension than the younger children. According to teachers' reports, all achievement abilities were found to improve over the initial 6-month recovery period, with less recovery seen 6 months to 2 years postinjury. Achievement testing showed average performance for all of the children 2 years after the injury. However, 79% of the severely injured children had either been retained in a grade or were receiving special education services. The investigators questioned the sensitivity of omnibus achievement tests for children with TBI. Jaffe and colleagues (1990) have suggested that difficulties in memory, visual–spatial ability, attention, and behavioral control may interact with school performance and account for the finding of age- and grade-appropriate achievement test scores in the face of failing school performance.

Although language deficits are reported to be present in many adults and children with TBI, it appears that receptive language skills are frequently spared following injury but expressive language skills are significantly affected. Ewing-Cobbs and colleagues (1987) have suggested that previously learned skills, such as the ability to comprehend language, are less susceptible to TBI than those emerging, such as the ability to express complex ideas. In addition, these researchers found that children with TBI showed significant difficulties in written language skills, particularly if the injury occurred during the 6- to 8-year-old period—an age believed to be when written language skills develop most rapidly (Levin et al., 1995). These same children experienced no difficulty in copying written language, thus ruling out a visual–motor deficit as the cause for the difficulties with written language. Such difficulties with expressive and written language are suggested to significantly disrupt the child's academic progress, particularly in reading and in written expression.

Bloom and colleagues (2000) evaluated children with TBI for long-term effects of difficulty in reading, spelling, and arithmetic. Children were separated into mild/moderate and severe groups for comparison. Significant long-term effects were found for reading, arithmetic, and spelling, the most significant weaknesses being present in children with the more severe injury. However, children with mild/moderate injury were also shown to evidence some impairment in all of these skills, although not to the degree shown in the severe TBI group. These deficits were found to persist at least 5 years from the time of injury.

Deficits in reading have been reported in the literature but are not well studied. Language difficulties have also been found but are generally of a subtle nature, including difficulties in understanding metaphors, drawing inferences, and formulating sentences (Dennis & Barnes, 1990). Disorganization in the process of expressing ideas or recalling information has been found in children with frontal lobe lesions (Chapman et al., 1992; Ylvisaker, 1998).

ATTENTION AND EXECUTIVE FUNCTIONING

Attention deficits are frequently seen following TBI and generally confound tests of memory. Although these two areas often interact on measures and in everyday life, they are discussed separately here for clarity's sake. Attentional difficulties also significantly disrupt long-term school achievement and emotional adjustment (Dennis et al., 1995). Attention is generally believed to consist of components involving alertness, sustained attention, divided attention, and selective attention (Sohlberg & Mateer, 1989). Attentional deficits are generally seen immediately following injury, but, for some children, resolve in the first year postinjury (Johnson & Roethig-Johnson, 1989; Van Zomeren & Brouwer, 1992). For others, attentional problems persist, mainly in the areas of sustained and selective attention, especially in children with severe head injuries (Kaufmann et al., 1993). Particular difficulty in the ability to focus, sustain, and shift attention has been found in young children with severe TBI (Ewing-Cobbs et al., 1998b).

Processing speed has been related to attentional deficits in several studies, which indicate that not only is attention an area of difficulty, but also the speed with which information is accessed (Catroppa et al., 1999).

Mittenberg and colleagues (1997) found that parents are more likely to report attentional difficulties than memory problems following a head injury. However, the attentional deficit was also related to the child's anxiety level and appeared to be part of a postconcussion syndrome rather than a full attentional deficit.

A long-term study by Dennis and colleagues (1995) found that a longer recovery time was associated with improvement in attention; that is, the more time that had elapsed from the occurrence of the head injury, the more recovery was seen in attentional tasks. This finding was true for older and younger children, although children who were younger when the injury occurred continued to experience attentional difficulties more than those injured at an older age. Additional findings included that children with TBI frequently showed difficulties with inhibition and with response modulation. Although selective attentional difficulties were found, these difficulties appeared to be more related to an inability to not attend to distractions. In other words, the children paid attention to everything and were easily distracted from the task at hand. When distractors were held to a minimum, the children showed adequate selective attention. Thus, it was the inability to focus on relevant detail that was particularly problematic for these children—not just selective attention.

These difficulties were more severely present in younger children, significantly compromising their ability to learn basic academic skills, whereas older children were more successful in inhibiting responses on tasks that they had mastered but not on novel tasks. Consistent with this finding, children with early head injury were later found to show a lower VIQ—such a finding indicates a difficulty in the storage and retrieval of knowledge (Dennis et al., 1995). Difficulty in sorting out important from unimportant information likely contributes to these academic and cognitive deficits. In addition, children with TBI were found to process the distractor as well as the target, thus using attentional capacity to process both stimuli.

Continuing difficulty with attention appears to be related to severe head injury, but not to mild or moderate head injury (Asarnow et al., 1995; Chadwick et al., 1981a). For children with mild or moderate head injury attentional problems have generally been found to resolve 2 years after the time of injury. However, in children younger than 5 at the time of the injury who sustain severe head trauma, the attentional deficits do not fully resolve.

Of additional concern is the finding that difficulties with executive functions are also frequently present in children with TBI (Begali, 1992; Lezak, 1994). These difficulties involve problems with planning and organization, as well as the child's insight into his/her own behavior. Such problems are frequently seen in the ability to generalize learning to similar situations, use rule-governed behavior, and use appropriate social behavior. Few studies have further elaborated this area, particularly on the relationship of deficits in executive functioning to MRI findings. One study evaluating the relationship of several measures of executive functions found correlations between measures of verbal fluency, inhibition, and perseveration, and frontal lobe lesions in the left hemisphere. Right frontal lesions were found in relationship to measures of semantic clustering, verbal fluency, and working memory (Levin et al., 1993, 1994).

MEMORY

Memory deficits are frequently found in children with TBI, particularly in the areas of verbal learning and verbal memory (Delis et al., 1994; Roman et al., 1998). In children with severe injuries difficulties persist and negatively affect their ability to learn and integrate new information. Hoffman and colleagues (2000) studied children with mild/moderate and severe head injuries on a measure of verbal learning, the California Verbal Learning Test—Children's Version (CVLT-C; Delis et al., 1994). Differences were found on this measure, with the children with severe head injuries performing the most poorly. When the individual indices of the CVLT-C were evaluated, no differences were found in measures of attention or in working memory. Differences were found on a measure of memory capacity, or the ability to learn with repetition.

The CVLT-C requires the examiner to repeat a word list five times. The children with severe head injuries did not show the same learning curve as those with mild head injuries, thus implying difficulty in maintaining information over time. Difficulties were also found in delayed recall and in the use of efficient learning strategies. This finding, which is consistent with that of Yeates and colleagues (1995; Yeates & Taylor, 1997), has implications for academic achievement. Thus, children with TBI may experience problems in accessing information that has been previously learned.

Similar difficulties were found by Nichols and colleagues (2000) using the CVLT-C. In this study children with perinatal focal brain lesions were found to perform more poorly than controls, particularly on tasks requiring immediate recall, consistency of recall, and progress over repetitions. No difference was found between the children with right versus left focal lesions—both groups experienced significant difficulty on these tasks. Conclusions from this study included the finding that early focal lesions significantly compromise the child's ability to remember verbal information over time and to develop new learning. Moreover, children were found to differ from adults in these abilities, as adults with left hemispheric lesions show more significant difficulty on these tasks than those with right hemispheric lesions. Thus, developmental issues are important variables in understanding children with TBI.

MRI scans have demonstrated lesions in the frontal lobes and temporal poles in children with memory difficulties (Levin et al., 1995, 1996). These findings suggest that the ability to store information and to organize it for later use is compromised in these children. Levin and colleagues (1995) suggest that additional damage is likely, particularly in the temporal lobes, but these lesions are not visible through MRI. The use of functional MRI techniques was suggested to document the extent of frontal lobe dysfunction on the functioning of additional brain regions such as the temporal lobes.

Working memory is the ability to hold information in your mind while performing a mental operation on it. For example, when you look up a phone number, you may rehearse the number while you are dialing it. Another example is the performance of a mental calculation, a task similar to the one on the arithmetic subtest of the WISC-III. Working memory is generally of short duration, and it requires rehearsal to maintain the information for more than a few seconds. Children with TBI have been found to show deficits in working memory, and recovery from these deficits appears to be sensitive to the severity of the injury, age at injury, and length of time from occurrence of the injury. Dennis and colleagues (2000) evaluated children with mild, moderate, and severe TBI on a measure of auditory-verbal working memory. Each child was required to remember words over a period of 3 to 24 seconds and then compare the initial words with new words. Working memory deficits were found for children with moderate to severe TBI, but not for those with mild TBI. The children with severe TBI showed the poorest performance, and this deficit persisted following recovery. Length of time from injury was not found to be related to working memory deficits, and age was related only for the severe TBI group. Recommendations included allowing additional time for tasks requiring working memory and educational support for these children.

PERCEPTUAL/VISUAL–MOTOR FUNCTIONING

Consistent with the aforementioned findings of compromised PIQ, many children with TBI also experience perceptual and visual–motor deficits. Manifestations of these difficulties may range from distortions of figures to be copied to an inability to integrate the figures. For example, on the Developmental Test of Visual–Motor Integration (VMI; Beery, 1990) one of the figures to be copied is a horizontal line bisected by an X. Children may be able to draw the lines in isolation, but they often have difficulty in integrating them. The Block Design subtest also provides information about configuration difficulties. Some children with TBI will confuse the internal configuration and reproduce a figure incorrectly. Such difficulties are associated with parietal lobe dysfunction (Lezak, 1994). Others experience difficulty with the outer configuration and fail to use a square in replicating the design; this difficulty is hypothesized to be attributable to frontal lobe dysfunction.

Children and adolescents with TBI have shown difficulties on the Bender–Gestalt test and on the Block Design subtest of the WISC-III. Difficulties with visual details, poor fine motor dexterity, and difficulty with analysis and synthesis have also been reported in children with TBI (Chadwick et al., 1981a, 1981b; Levin & Eisenberg, 1979; Lezak, 1994; Luria, 1980). Difficulties with visual–motor tasks appear to be compounded when a time element is introduced, as in the PIQ (Bowden et al., 1985). These problems are especially prominent in children with severe head injury, particularly those under 12 years of age (Levin et al., 1995).

PSYCHOSOCIAL AND BEHAVIORAL FUNCTIONING

Behavioral and psychosocial difficulties are fairly common in children with TBI (DiScala et al., 1991), and these problems cause parents and teachers the greatest distress (Levin, 1987). Jaffe and colleagues (1990) suggest that there are two categories of psychosocial and behavioral difficulties. Problems of the first category occur during the initial stage of recovery and involve behaviors that are transient. Agitation, poor verbal understanding, and regressive behaviors are frequently seen, which quickly resolve with a child's regaining consciousness and orientation. During this period of time subtle cognitive deficits, awareness of the injury and resulting depression, and low self-esteem are also present. Behavioral difficulties of the second category are more permanent and have been reported in several studies. Premorbid functioning is predictive of postmorbid functioning, as discussed in earlier chapters. Such premorbid functioning, coupled with the severity of the injury and the reactions of the child and the family to the injury, may provide a helpful model for understanding the variability of outcomes following TBI. Children with premorbid behavioral and emotional difficulties coupled with fewer social supports appear to fare more poorly then those with intact families and better preinjury functioning. There appears to be an overrepresentation of children with premorbid behavioral difficulties who come from chaotic or disruptive family backgrounds (Jaffe et al., 1990). This finding has implications for the support of the child, as well as for the outcome.

Behaviors reported by parents to be especially worrisome include inattention, hyperactivity, and irritability. Low tolerance for frustration and poor motivation have also been reported (McAllister, 1992; Michaud et al., 1993). Difficulty with anger modulation, aggressive behavior, anxiety, and depression, as well as a tendency for a child to socially isolate him/herself and to use various substances for self-medication are also reported to be particularly distressing for caretakers (Kehle et al., 1996). Early expression of irritability has been found to be related to the later development of aggressive behavior (McKinlay et al., 1981; Silver & Yudofsky, 1987). These difficulties do not appear to resolve as quickly as motor and visual–spatial deficits and often persist for an extended period of time. When psychosocial and emotional difficulties are accompanied by an underlying cognitive component (inability to learn from behaviors, memory deficits, and/or attentional difficulties), they are more difficult to remediate and take significantly more time to resolve (DiScala et al., 1991). Additional variables that may relate to the ability to resolve such difficulties range from the number of parents in the household to the age of the child in a single-parent home (younger children experience more difficulties and poorer outcomes) (Tompkins et al., 1990).

Psychosocial and behavioral difficulties are particularly worrisome, because these problems can affect academic and cognitive progress and later social competence (Rosenthal & Bond, 1990). For example, cognitive deficits have been found to affect the acquisition of social skills in children who experienced TBI prior to age 7 (Ewing-Cobbs et al., 2000). Children who experienced TBI as a result of child abuse were found to show more indications of negative affect than those with TBI not due to child abuse. Infants and preschoolers with abuse-inflicted TBI have also been found to show poorer adaptive behavior following recovery (Prasad et al., 2000). Thus, for children with TBI due to child abuse, it appears that the caretaker–child relationship is even more predictive of poor outcome than the injury itself. Family factors are important in rehabilitation and are discussed more fully in Chapter 4.

Children with TBI have been shown to evidence hyperarousal and frustration, with many showing more headaches and stomachaches than those with non-TBI injuries (Vriezen, 2000). The incidence of depression has been found to be increased in this population; symptoms show poor resolution, particularly in children with severe TBI and, to a lesser extent, in children with moderate TBI (Janusz et al., 2000). These difficulties have been found to persist more than a year following the injury.

Posttraumatic stress symptoms have also been identified in children with TBI. Levi and colleagues (1999) studied children aged 6 to 12 who had sustained TBI or orthopedic injury (OI). Children with severe TBI showed higher levels of posttraumatic stress symptoms then those with mild TBI or OI. Follow-up at 6 months and at 1 year found these symptoms continuing in degree and frequency. Ethnicity and age at injury were not related to posttraumatic symptoms, but socioeconomic status (SES) was—children of lower SES showed more stress.

The suggestion that children with TBI will show social difficulties is consistent with the preceding findings for the persistence of depressive and anxiety symptoms, as well as the likelihood that younger children will experience difficulty in developing social competence. Some researchers have suggested that children with TBI may show a deterioration in social skills over time because of an awareness of previously obtained but now lost skills (Begali, 1992; Fordyce et al., 1983). This hypothesis has not been carefully studied and should be viewed as a clinical observation rather than as an expectation.

Self-awareness deficits have also been found, as well as difficulty with the development of insight (Thomsen, 1984). Younger children may not be accepted by former friends and may resort to social withdrawal or aggressive behaviors. There is evidence that children with TBI have difficulty with social communication skills, which further affects their friendships and peer interactions (Ylvisaker, 1993). For adolescents, difficulties with identity formation and independence may become stumbling blocks to further development.

Substance abuse is an area of particular concern with adolescents. The use of alcohol by adolescents with TBI has been documented in the literature, with reviews suggesting that one-third to one-half of head injury patients were intoxicated at the time of the injury (Corrigan, 1995; Rimel et al., 1982). Kreutzer and colleagues (1996) studied adolescents with TBI aged 16 to 20. Preinjury drinking did not differ between these adolescents and age-matched controls. Males showed more drinking behavior than females in both the TBI and control groups. At the initial follow-up after the injury (2 to 15 months postinjury), substance abuse was decreased as compared with preinjury use. These findings were also present in the second follow-up period (16 to 47 months postinjury). However, those patients who had been heavy drinkers prior to their injuries showed significant drinking at the second follow-up visit, as well as an increase in drinking as compared with the first follow-up visit. By the second follow-up visit 44% fell within the moderate-to-heavy drinker category. Thus, substance abuse prior to the accident was strongly predictive of substance abuse postinjury.

In a study of adolescents and young adults with TBI, TBI and substance abuse, and substance abuse alone, MRI findings showed consistent group differences, with the TBI group as a whole showing degenerative changes after the trauma. However, the TBI-plus-substance-abuse group showed the most atrophy on all morphometric measures (Barker et al., 1999). The finding that the TBI-plus-substance-abuse group showed more neuroanatomical damage may reflect the likelihood of patients who are intoxicated to be at higher risk for additional neurological damage, resulting from the increased permeability of the blood–brain barrier at the time of the accident (Kelly, 1995; Kelly et al., 1997). Neuropsychologically, all groups did poorly, and there were no significant differences between the groups. However, there was a trend for the TBI-plus-substance-abuse group to perform the most poorly. Thus, substance abuse at all times (before, during, and after a TBI incident) places the adolescent at higher risk of long-term damage and poorer outcome. Substance abuse is an important variable to consider when an adolescent is evaluated for appropriate programming and educational remediation.

Richard, the adolescent introduced in Chapter 1, showed difficulty in the area of attention and memory. Prior to the accident he had been an A/B student with a circle of friends. He participated in football and was on the starting team. Following the accident, Richard's friends initially visited him and provided support. As he began to recover and physically showed no lasting effects, his friends came to see him less often. He experienced difficulty in relating to his peers, was labile in mood, and had difficulty with disinhibition.

Homeschooling during this period was somewhat problematic, as he experienced fatigue when working for more than 2 hours, had difficulty retaining material from the previous lesson, and had a very short fuse. His tolerance for frustration was markedly lower than prior to the accident, and he found himself in frequent conflict with his mother. Richard's affect alternated from quite argumentative to sad and withdrawn.

Upon reentrance to school Richard initially seemed happier and better adjusted. He began football practice with his team and experienced slight difficulty with attention on the football field. Academically, Richard was struggling in the regular classroom and yet reluctant to take advantage of the special education support provided to him. He rarely asked for assistance and by midterm was failing most of his classes. He continued to participate in peer activities but had moved from a leadership role to one more characteristic of a follower. Prior to the accident his peer relationships had been satisfying, but Richard was no longer sought out by his peers for social activities. He wasn't excluded from group activities, but just not encouraged to participate as much as he had been prior to the TBI.

Richard became more argumentative at home and resistant to rules and routines. He was dropped from the football team because of arguing with the coach. His frequent arguments with his mother were such that Richard's father had to physically intervene at times. Richard's affect ranged generally from withdrawn to depressed. His parents were very worried about him, both emotionally and cognitively, and requested an evaluation of his skills to determine how best to meet his needs. Richard reluctantly agreed to such an assessment, although he adamantly denied that anything was "wrong" with him.

The family can affect a child's recovery, as can the support provided by the school and other community agencies. It is important to understand the stresses the family experiences during a child's recovery from TBI. The following chapter discusses these concerns in more detail.

CHAPTER 4

♦♦♦

Family Influences on
Children and Adolescents

♦

As in Richard's case (introduced in Chapter 1), the family contributes greatly to the outcome of TBI and the recovery of the child or adolescent. Initially, in cases of severe injury and/or illnesses, the family's first concern is the survival of the child (Semrud-Clikeman, 1999). When survival is assured, questions are raised as to the eventual functioning of the patient. If the patient's functioning is significantly compromised, the family members go through a grieving process quite similar to that experienced when there is a death in the family (Brooks, 1990). When families are unable to cope with such difficulties, the outcome is significantly compromised and behavioral problems are generally exacerbated (Taylor et al., 1995). Research on the role of the family in TBI recovery is not extensive; the few studies available point to the family environment as a variable in eventual recovery (Brooks, 1991).

Families go through stages during the recovery of a child or adolescent. Physical concerns are initially paramount and given the most attention. As the child's motor and sensory skills resolve, deficits in behavioral and cognitive skills become more important and may be far more challenging (Allen et al., 1994; Fletcher et al., 1990). Improvements frequently occur fairly rapidly in the first 6 to 12 months following the accident. Thereafter, however, recovery becomes much slower and parental frustration follows—this is the beginning of the grieving process (Rosenthal & Muir, 1983; Semrud-Clikeman, 1999). When the child begins to miss expected developmental milestones (such as getting a driver's license), the distress of the parents and family may rekindle their sense that the child, as known previously, has not survived (Semrud-Clikeman, 1999). In fact, some researchers refer to these children as "almosters" (Jackson & Haverkamp,

1991). Conoley and Sheridan (1996) describe this concept as the child who is almost the same as before, but in many important ways is not the same—such a difference can lead to depression and anxiety about the child's future.

Among the areas of frequent concern in families are financial hardship following the injury and the adjustment required, not only by parents but also by siblings. In addition, the degree of cohesiveness in the family and the communication patterns appear to be predictive of eventual outcome (DePompei & Zarski, 1989). Thus, support provided by health professionals and school personnel is needed to assist the family as a whole to cope with the injury. Social support and help with transitions between the various institutions (hospital to home to school) are important in assisting the child in the recovery process (Waaland & Kreutzer, 1991).

When families have been studied approximately 1 year after an injury, Harris and colleagues (1989) found that the majority of the marriages became problematic and more than 65% reported difficulty with siblings. Siblings have been found to experience considerable conflict in their feelings toward the injured family member. Generally, significant amounts of attention are provided to the injured child, frequently at the expense of the other siblings. Although such attention is certainly merited, the siblings are likely to experience feelings of jealousy, anger, and anxiety, particularly if the recovery is of long duration. Some investigators have found that siblings may attempt to gain the attention of their parents, at the same time feeling guilty about their own needs for affection (Dyson et al., 1989; Simeonsson & Bailey, 1986). These difficulties have been found to be present more than 5 years after the injury and are compounded by the siblings' feeling that they can "never live up to" the injury the child has experienced (Orsillo et al., 1993). There is some documentation that such siblings are at higher risk for development of behavioral problems and affective disorders (Breslau, 1982, 1983). Moreover, it is suggested that younger males experience more difficulty than female siblings and those who are not close in age to the injured family member (Conoley & Sheridan, 1996)

Hu and colleagues (1993) found that when the mother was suffering from a psychological disorder (i.e., depression/anxiety) in families in which a child had experienced either a significant illness or TBI, the child's behavior was poorer than when the mother's mental health was intact. Single-parent homes were found to be at highest risk for disruption and poorer outcome. Very little study has been conducted to evaluate the TBI family exclusively. As discussed earlier, there have been findings that premorbid behavioral disturbances are predictive of difficulties after TBI, but few studies have evaluated the status of families prior to the injury as compared with disruption following the injury (Taylor et al., 1995). It is likely that the families who experienced difficulty prior to the injury are at higher risk of dissolution or disruption following such an accident.

A few studies have evaluated the TBI family and found that parents report more stress in their marriage, more difficulty with the child/adolescent with TBI than with the siblings, and more depressive parental symptoms (Perrott et al., 1991). When severity of injury was added to the evaluation, families with children with severe injury showed more disruption in functioning than families of children with mild or moderate injury (Rivara et al., 1992). In addition, family functioning prior to the injury was seen as highly predictive of later difficulties, with the less cohesive and more chaotic families showing the poorest adjustment (Rivara et al., 1993; Wade et al., 1995). Most children who achieve cognitive recovery have been found to show persistent behavioral and adaptive behavior problems, particularly in families that are disruptive and noncohesive and in which communication patterns are poor (Boll, 1983; Fletcher et al., 1990; Perrott et al., 1991).

Taylor and colleagues (1995) studied families of children with TBI and compared them with families of children with orthopedic injury. The children with TBI experienced moderate to severe TBI and were aged 6 to 12 years at the time of injury. Procedures included parent interviews and ratings, teacher ratings of preinjury behavior, and review of each child's medical chart. Tests for depression, academic achievement and IQ, psychomotor skills, language, memory and attention, and executive functioning were conducted once the child was medically stabilized. Both groups showed family stress following the injuries. Preliminary data analysis indicated that the TBI group experienced more enduring difficulties than families of children with orthopedic injuries. There were also findings that higher rates of child behavior problems were associated with more family disruption, greater parental psychopathology, and poorer family functioning. Conclusions drawn from this ongoing study suggest that interventions are required for the best possible outcomes and that environmental factors may be as predictive of rehabilitation success as the nature of the injury itself.

Wade and colleagues (1996) sought to identify the factors distinguishing those families that cope well with TBI from those that do not. Families and their children with moderate to severe TBI were compared with families and children with orthopedic injuries. Families of children with severe TBI were found to experience the most stress as compared with the families of children with moderate TBI and those with orthopedic injuries. As compared with the moderate TBI and orthopedic groups, the severe TBI group showed more stress in interactions with other family members (siblings and grandparents) and heightened levels of anxiety. Areas of particular concern included worries about the child's recovery and a more frequent tendency for parents with children with severe TBI to request assistance with child care, housekeeping services, and financial assistance. Counseling and emotional assistance were infrequently mentioned or requested by families with children with any type of injury. This finding is particularly important, as the families were experiencing significant emotional distress, and yet, when asked what they needed, requested more concrete forms of assistance (housekeeping, financial). Wade and colleagues recommend that parents be provided with information about the stresses and emotional concerns that will arise with TBI, and guidance for coping with these feelings. When provided with such services, the parents in this study reported relief and appreciation of the ability to discuss their anxieties with a concerned professional.

Conoley and Sheridan (1996) suggest that families of children with TBI experience two types of burdens: objective and subjective. Objective burdens include the child's neuropsychological and cognitive deficits, and subjective burdens are those concerning the level of distress experienced by family members. Subjective burdens are reported to fall more heavily on mothers and are more predictive of family distress than objective burdens (Allen et al., 1994). These burdens have been found to increase over time, with divorce, substance abuse, and social isolation appearing to be possible outcomes (Brooks et al., 1986, 1987; Conoley & Sheridan, 1996). Emotional responses in mothers have been found to include frustration, anger, lability, depression, and overprotection (Brooks, 1991; Mauss-Clum & Ryan, 1981).

Interventions that families report to be most helpful include information about the child's health, educational programs available to the child, and community agencies available for assistance (Miller, 1993). A concern is that parents may develop an adversarial relationship with health professionals, stemming from disillusionment with the child's progress and frustration in dealing with various systems in the child's life (hospital, rehabilitation center, rehabilitation specialists). These difficulties have been found to carry over into relationships with school personnel and may color these interactions as well (Martin, 1988). Thus, it is particularly important that school personnel be aware of the stresses a family is experiencing, particularly as Individualized Educational Plans (IEPs) and special education services are being developed.

INTERVENTIONS

One of the most important aspects of interventions with families is the provision of current and practical information about their children's progress, disabilities, and educational needs. Understandable information about a child's injury and the nature of his/her deficits is important. This information may need to be repeated frequently, with additional details and depth provided as the child recovers. Yet too many details or too much information at one time may only confuse rather than provide assistance (Lezak, 1988). For example, recall an experience with medical or school personnel when you were given bad news. For most of us, when we become upset or anxious, it is quite hard to focus on what is being said. Frequently, a doctor or school professional will continue talking about the problem, giving details and opinions, not observing that the patient/parent is now overwhelmed and unable to absorb the information being given. Unfortunately, this state of affairs is particularly likely when a parent is still quite upset about the injury and the professional continues to talk about the injury. It is more appropriate to provide information in small bits and to answer the questions the parents have at the time. In most cases, school personnel do not see the child at this point, but when they do talk with parents, it will be important to keep in mind that parents who are anxious or concerned about the child's schooling can be unable to absorb information at this point as well. It will be important for professionals to provide more than one opportunity for the parent to talk about the child's needs and for school personnel to explain the resources available to the child and parent.

Meetings including large numbers of people can be quite intimidating and overwhelming for some parents. It is important that a premeeting be arranged to discuss major findings with parents and to explain the individuals who will attend these meetings. A discussion of the roles of the physical therapist, the occupational therapist, and the speech pathologist can help smooth the way for a productive meeting.

The IEP is recommended as a tool to assist the parent in understanding what will be required of his/her child, as well as the school's expectations of the parent (Conoley & Sheridan, 1996). It is particularly important for the school psychologist/counselor to be versed in the injury sustained by the child and to be able to translate these difficulties into educational and social recommendations. The school psychologist is in a particularly good position to provide such translation and to be sensitive to the parent's needs and ability to absorb information about school resources. It is important to recall Conoley and Sheridan's (1996) suggestion that the parent's subjective burden appears to *increase* over time and that the IEP may trigger feelings of frustration and anger about the injury and the loss of the child.

Lezak (1988) suggests that it is important for parents to be aware that recovery is not an all-or-none process. Some skills may be recovered fairly rapidly, whereas others may not reappear quickly or at all. Moreover, parents may have to be provided respite from the child's needs and must look after their own emotional health. As described earlier in this chapter, parents are at high risk for the development of affective disorders; marital discord, and even divorce, may occur. It is also important for the parent to recognize that the child may resist some of the assistance provided and may confront the parent, thus adding to the parent's discomfort.

Richard, the adolescent introduced in Chapter 1, continually fought against his parents' restrictions and became quite angry when not allowed to drive the family car. These confrontations became increasingly frequent and resulted in the family's requiring therapy to assist in the development of rules and expectations that met both Richard's and his parents' needs. A number of issues were important subjects for discussion, such as Richard's development of independent skills and his anger over losing some of the privileges he had previously enjoyed (driving a car was prevented by the possibility of seizures). In addition, his parents had to come to terms with their natural tendency to overprotect Richard and shelter him from the disappointments that were inevitable during recovery.

COMMUNITY AGENCIES

The availability of community agencies is an important variable in working with families of children with TBI. Legal and financial concerns become more salient. Involvement in the legal system generally places further stress on a family that is a defendant or a plaintiff in a lawsuit. It is important for the child's school to be aware of such additional stressors. It is likely that the school psychologist will be asked by an attorney or a community agency about the child's progress and the programs available to the child. A case manager from a rehabilitation center or a community agency may also be available to assist the parent in finding helpful resources and to provide guidance through the family's financial and emotional stresses. Case management can also help by coordinating the services of the various agencies.

As in Richard's case, family therapy is frequently warranted. Often, this intervention is not attempted until a situation has become very difficult for all involved (Conoley & Sheridan, 1996). Such therapy can assist the injured child/adolescent, siblings, and parents to explore how the family has changed, the positive aspects that remain in the family, and the negative behaviors that may be polarizing family members. In addition, various coping mechanisms the family may have used previously may be adapted to reflect the changed family environment. The incorporation of new behaviors by all family members must be stressed, rather than simply the change in the brain-injured child. Thinking of the family as a system that has been irrevocably changed may assist in the reorganization necessary for the family unit to survive.

In Richard's case, he had been the sibling his younger brothers looked up to and from whom they expected help. To his parents, he had been a reliable adolescent who could be trusted to fulfill his obligations. Following his head injury, Richard had more difficulty fulfilling these obligations and, in practical terms, had problems in doing more than one activity at a time. For example, when asked to watch his 7-year-old sister, Richard became distracted by working on a task, and his sister wandered off. She was found, unharmed, at a neighbor's house three doors down from the family home. It was important in the family session to assist his parents in changing their expectations and to help Richard cope with the loss of self-esteem he experienced in light of his changed abilities.

National organizations can also provide support to families in need. The National Head Injury Foundation can be quite helpful in providing additional information. Support groups may be helpful as well, and it is possible that information about these groups can be obtained through a local hospital or rehabilitation center. Additional resources are provided in Table 4.1.

HOME–SCHOOL PARTNERSHIPS

When a child/adolescent reenters school following a head injury (or other serious illness), it is of paramount importance that a partnership be formed between the parents and the school personnel. Such a partnership is only begun with the development of the IEP, and, as discussed in Chapter 5, the

TABLE 4.1. Family Resources

Organization	Address	Phone
Brain Injury Association	1776 Massachusetts Avenue NW Suite 100 Washington, DC 20036	1-800-444-6443
National Rehabilitation Information Center	8455 Colesville Road, #935 Silver Spring, MD 20910	1-800-346-2742
National Information Center for Children and Youth with Handicaps	P.O. Box 1492 Washington, DC 20013	1-800-999-5599
National Center for Youth with Disabilities	Adolescent Health Program University of Minnesota Box 721-UMHC Minneapolis, MN 55455	1-800-333-NCYD
National Neurobehavioral Resource Center		1-800-775-NNRC
Pediatric Brain Injury Resource Center	230 South 500 East, #100 Salt Lake City, UT 84102	
National Head Injury Foundation		1-800-444-NHIF

child's needs will change, as will the IEP, and, ultimately, so will the home–school partnership. It is important to build bridges at the beginning of this association, and the role of the school psychologist and/or school practitioner is central to the relationship. Many of the techniques used during the school day must be translated into use at home, and therapies such as occupational therapy, speech and language therapy, and physical therapy require home programs for maximum effectiveness. Open communication between home and school is always important, but particularly so for children with TBI. Behaviors that may be problematic at home may not be seen at school or vice versa.

Sara, a 7-year-old child who experienced a severe skull fracture and neurosurgery for a hematoma, was able to maintain her emotional balance during a shortened school day of 5 hours. However, once she arrived home, she became extremely irritable, was difficult to discipline, and was very tired. Communication between home and school brought these behaviors to the attention of her teacher. It was agreed that the 5-hour school day was too taxing and that expectations should be altered. The little girl was provided an opportunity for a short nap at midmorning to regain her strength and her day was thus shortened. This small change resulted in a smoother transition between home and school.

Conoley and Sheridan (1996) have presented a model for home–school partnerships, which they have labeled an *empowerment model.* This model's basic tenet is that the family and the school join together in the identification of problems and their solutions. Parents are seen as an integral part of the relationship and as active problem solvers. This model differs from the medical model whereby the professional tells the patient what has happened and what to do and the patient complies with medical advice. The Conoley and Sheridan model suggests a collaborative relationship in which neither party is superior, with particular emphasis on the strengths of both the family and the school. The IEP becomes a working document that incorporates needed changes as the child grows and is also a means of communication for both parties. In addition, the plan is dynamic in that it changes with the demands placed on the child and the resulting problems that can arise.

The model suggests four stages, beginning with problem identification. In this phase one or two issues are identified as paramount and information is gathered concerning these issues (Sheridan et al., 1996). Sara, the 7-year-old child described earlier, provides an illustration of how these stages can be implemented. First, it was determined that her difficult behavior occurred shortly after she arrived home from school and did not happen on weekends. Second, a journal was developed to document the behaviors, including what had happened just prior to the behavior and the consequences of the behavior. Thus, the behaviors were pinpointed as to their frequency and time of occurrence. Evaluation of this journal indicated that Sara's difficult behaviors occurred before lunch but never after her nap. In addition, the journal reflected the mother's subjective concern, as she watched her child come from the bus stop, that the afternoon may be quite difficult. The journal also provided information about what had occurred in the morning at school, particularly right before Sara was dismissed.

In the second stage, problem analysis (Kratochwill & Bergan, 1990), the data are discussed, including what occurs just prior to the behavior and the consequences of the behavior. For Sara, the area of concern that emerged was her fatigue resulting from the 5-hour day. It is not uncommon for children with severe TBI to experience fatigue more easily than they did prior to injury. In this case the school psychologist was able to relate Sara's difficulties with her current behavior. In addition, it was discovered that Sara was being teased by her peers about leaving school early. This finding indicated additional social stresses of which both her teacher and her parents had been unaware. Moreover, Sara's mother discovered that her anxiety increased as the time for Sara to return home approached, making her a bit more edgy when Sara came through the door. When Sara became upset, her mother found herself yelling at her daughter rather than being able to calmly deal with the child's concerns.

In the third stage, a plan is developed for both the school and the parents to assist with the behavioral changes. First, Sara's school day was further shortened to 4 hours, with a nap provided midmorning. Second, Sara's peers were counseled about her needs and how the teasing was making her feel. Third, Sara's mother offered some suggestions as to how she might better cope with her daughter's demands and irritability when she became more fatigued. Helping Sara's mother to realize that most of Sara's behaviors were not willful but a result of her TBI appeared to somewhat allay the anxiety involved in this interaction.

Finally, in the fourth stage, the success of the program is evaluated by all parties. In Sara's case, a meeting of the teacher, school psychologist, and parents indicated that most of the plan was working well. It was decided that Sara's day would remain at 4 hours until her fatigue appeared to resolve and would gradually return to the 5 hours originally scheduled.

CONCLUSION

It is very important to recognize the stresses on the family unit when a child or adolescent has suffered TBI. The more severe the injury, the heavier the stress load. It is also important to recognize the contribution of prior difficulties in the adjustment of the family to the injury. Families that have experienced significant discord and stress in the past are likely to be in danger of experiencing greater difficulty after the injury. Conversely, families with good communication and cohesiveness generally provide their members with good social support. Emerging research suggests that the main predictor for a good outcome may not be the nature of injury itself, but rather the environment in which the child finds him/herself following such injury. Just as premorbid behavioral and personality disturbances have been found to be predictive of similar problems after an injury, family discord prior to an injury is highly predictive of divorce, social isolation, and substance abuse following a child's TBI.

Home–school partnerships are particularly important for a smooth transition to the school setting. In addition, these partnerships allow for an adjustment of the IEP and carryover of the various therapies many of the children require. The medical model of the expert telling the patient what to do is not appropriate for working with children with TBI in the school. Rather, when a partnership is forged, all members of the team benefit. The use of conjoint consultation to assist with problem resolution is particularly important. The child's needs are dynamic and ever changing, and such a partnership allows for the adjustment of techniques that may not be optimal. These partnerships evolve over time, and with care and nurturing provide a safety net for the child and direction for future requirements.

The following chapter discusses the neuropsychological evaluation of various functional systems. A case is presented in detail at the end of the chapter. There are also suggestions as to assessment instruments that school personnel can utilize to further evaluate a child's need for comprehensive neuropsychological evaluation.

CHAPTER 5

◆◆◆

Neuropsychological Assessment

◆

Children and adolescents who have experienced TBI require a comprehensive neuropsychological evaluation, particularly if the level of injury is in the moderate-to-severe range. Such evaluations are frequently accomplished during the child's hospital stay and provide a baseline for recovery. A neuropsychological evaluation generally involves assessment of the child's functioning in a number of domains, including visual–spatial, perceptual, kinesthetic, working memory, executive functions, memory, attention, cognitive, and academic. In addition, a comprehensive neuropsychological evaluation will include measures of emotional and behavioral functioning. Such evaluations are not only useful to measure recovery of function but also to evaluate treatment efficiency (Coutts et al., 1987). Schools are now mandated to provide services to children with TBI who meet criteria for placement. Laws including Public Law 101-476 (Individuals with Disabilities Education Act [IDEA], Federal Register, 1990) and Section 504 of the Rehabilitation Act of 1973 require modifications of a child's educational program when services are warranted.

THE APPLICATION OF THE IDEA AND SECTION 504 TO TRAUMATIC BRAIN INJURY

Children and adolescents with TBI are covered under the IDEA and its recent revision. As school practitioners are aware, the IDEA provides a free and appropriate education for children and adolescents aged 3 to 21 with one or more of several disabling conditions. In the past children with TBI could be classified for services under one of the existing categories, including learning disability, mental retardation, other health impaired, emotionally disturbed, and physically handicapped. Under the original Public Law 94-142 (Federal Register, 1975), a minority, but sizable number, of children with TBI would not qualify for services even when such special education services were appropriate (Harrington, 1990). When Public Law 94-142 was revised, the category of TBI was recognized and became a fundable category (Russell, 1993).

The educational definition for TBI as set by the Code of Federal Regulations Part 300 (1993) is as follows:

> An acquired injury to the brain caused by an external physical force, resulting in total or partial functional disability or psychosocial impairment, or both that adversely affects a child's educational performance. The term applies to open or closed head injuries resulting in impairments in one or more areas, such as cognition; language; memory; attention; reasoning; abstract thinking; judgment; problem solving; sensory, perceptual, and motor abilities; psychosocial behavior; physical functions; information processing; and speech. The term does not apply to brain injuries that are congenital or degenerative, or brain injuries induced by birth trauma. (p. 14)

As can be seen from this definition, assessment of TBI is particularly relevant for school personnel. Although an initial neuropsychological evaluation may have occurred prior to reentry into school, many children do not have routinely scheduled follow-up neuropsychological evaluations. Best practices would include serial evaluations of these children's progress. In a survey of school psychology training programs, Walker and colleagues (1999) found that although school psychologists are in a primary position for assessing and developing intervention programs for children with TBI, most training programs do not offer training in assessment of these children. Thus, most school psychologists are not well prepared to develop programs for them.

With development, children may show skills that emerge (or do not emerge) as would be expected, with damage to particular areas not in evidence until a particular developmental skill is expected to emerge. An IEP is a dynamic document that changes with the child's development, and periodic assessment of children with TBI is important. For a child with TBI who appears to have reached a plateau in recovery or whose skills appear to be regressing, referral for a comprehensive evaluation is particularly relevant. However, even for those children continuing to make progress, it is important for school personnel and, most especially, the school psychologist to continue to monitor and evaluate such progress.

ASSESSMENT

The initial assessment of a child with TBI is quite complex as (1) multiple difficulties are frequently seen, (2) brain injuries to the same location may result in different skill deficits in different children, (3) recovery is complex and related to environmental factors, and (4) few tests have been developed and standardized specifically for TBI (Harrington, 1990). Moreover, as discussed in Chapter 3, the areas most frequently affected by TBI include attention, memory, language, cognitive skills, and emotional/behavioral functioning. Educators must be aware of the variance in symptoms shown by children with TBI and the appropriate measures to evaluate such difficulties.

An assessment of a child's skill levels must include standardized as well as informal measures. One of the more important methods is to evaluate the child's response to environmental demands both in the classroom and during the testing session. It is particularly important to pay attention to the child's ability to adapt to changing classroom routines. Additional areas to be evaluated include (1) attention span, (2) frustration tolerance, (3) fatigue, (4) need for routine, (5) confusion as to what is expected of him/her, (6) amount of time required for the child to process information, (7) how the child learns new material, (8) consistency of performance, and (9) learning strategies utilized (Harrington, 1990). Each of these areas provides information as to the child's ability to perform at the present time. In addition to obtaining these observations and teacher reports, it is important to gather information as to the child's premorbid functioning.

It is often the case that psychological evaluations have not been conducted prior to a child's injury. However, standardized test scores, report cards, and developmental information can be gathered to provide a marker for the child's previous level of performance. It is important to determine the child's prior strengths and weaknesses, not only to establish a blueprint for possible recovery of these skills, but also to assist the child, family, and school in generating realistic goals and plans for future development.

In addition to ascertaining the child's previous level of functioning, it is important for school personnel to obtain medical records relating to the child's injury. Particularly important is information as to the location of the injury, length of coma or loss of consciousness, and length of posttraumatic amnesia (Harrington, 1990). Information about medications that have been prescribed as well as medical concerns that have been raised should also be obtained. School personnel, including the school psychologist, school nurse, occupational therapist, physical therapist, and speech pathologist should be informed of these findings to assist in assessment of the child's needs. A suggested developmental questionnaire is presented in Table 5.1.

Assessment of children and young adolescents for central nervous system (CNS) dysfunction is more difficult than that of older adolescents and adults. The correlation between test results and CNS damage is not as well understood for children as for adults, and inferences about such relationships must be made only with firm evidence (Rutter, 1981; Taylor et al., 1984). A

TABLE 5.1. Sample Developmental Questionnaire

Whom does the child live with?

Parents' education and current occupations

Ages and sex of siblings

Who takes care of the child most of the time? Whom would the child approach if in trouble?

Description of pregnancy
- Any medications taken during pregnancy?
- Alcohol, tobacco, or other substances used during pregnancy?
- X-rays during pregnancy? Why?
- Maternal illnesses during pregnancy?
- What was the mother's emotional state during pregnancy?
- Did the mother experience toxemia, swelling, excessive weight gain? If yes, circle.

Birth history
- Length of pregnancy
- Length of labor
- Apgar score
- Birth weight
- Any problems after birth? Jaundice? Incubator? Breathing problems?

Developmental history
- Age child sat alone, crawled, walked, used first words, spoke in sentences.
- Age child toilet trained—day; night.
- Describe the child's early temperament. Did the child sleep through the night? Eating habits, soothability, need for routine.

Medical history
- Childhood illnesses (measles, mumps, chicken pox, etc.)
- Head injuries (duration of loss of consciousness, coma, hospitalization)
- Sustained high fever?
- Allergies
- Medications currently prescribed—how long and amount?
- Has the child had psychological counseling? Why and what type?
- Has the child had neuropsychological or psychological testing? Results?
- Has the child had a neurological workup? CT? MRI? Results?

Family history
- How many moves during the child's life? How many different schools?
- Family history of illnesses (learning disabilities, mental illness, ADHD).
- Divorce? What was the child's age?
- Remarriage? What was the child's age? How did child accept the marriage?
- Stepsiblings? Relationships?

School history
- When did the child begin school?
- If the child attended preschool, any problems?
- At what age did the child attend kindergarten?
- Has the child repeated any grades? If so, what grade(s)?
- Has the child been tested psychologically or educationally?
- Has the child been enrolled in special education? If so, in what category?
- Does the child have difficulty in any academic area? Describe.

(continued)

TABLE 5.1. (*continued*)

Peer relationships/emotional history
- How does the child relate to his/her peers?
- Does the child have a best friend?
- What hobbies and activities does the child enjoy?
- What is the parents' goal for their child?

developing brain is organized differently than an adult brain, and the emphasis must be placed on the interrelationship between the measures rather than on the measures and hypothesized brain damage (Ylvisaker et al., 1990).

Thus, for an assessment to be fully useful it must evaluate the core domains of functioning, placing them within the developmental framework, as well as the level of skills the child had prior to the injury. Second, the assessment should be remediation based—that is, scores should be used to understand *how* the child learns as much as to understand *what* the child knows. Third, it is important to understand the child's strengths and weaknesses in order to develop appropriate intervention techniques. In addition, the strengths and weaknesses should be evaluated as to their effect on the child's overall functioning. A weakness in holding a pencil is less likely to be important for later adjustment as a child's inability to learn new material. Concurrently with determining the child's strengths and weaknesses, it is important to identify the motivational, emotional, and social variables that affect the child's level of functioning (Ylvisaker et al., 1990). Such variables may be highly predictive of the child's ability to use and benefit from a remediation program, even one that is well designed may not be successful if the child does not fully participate in the intervention. It is also important to determine whether the most appropriate route is remediation or compensation. A child who is older and in middle school may not benefit from a strong phonics program to remediate reading difficulties as much as a program assisting him/her to develop compensation techniques for learning. In contrast, a child in second grade may be most appropriately tutored in phonics for reading. Motivation can also determine the appropriateness of remediation versus compensation. A child who is not strongly motivated is not likely to participate readily in a program that is strong on drill and rote memory and short on interest. Adapting the program to the child is the most appropriate plan rather than seeking to adapt the child to the program.

THREE NEUROPSYCHOLOGICAL METHODS FOR ASSESSMENT

There are three recognized methods for evaluating children from a neuropsychological point of view: the Halstead batteries, the Luria–Nebraska Battery, and the Boston Process Approach. All of these techniques require extensive training and supervision and are generally beyond the level of the specialist in school psychology. However, it is helpful to understand what each of the batteries can and cannot measure.

Halstead–Reitan Batteries

The most frequently used neuropsychological battery (Howieson & Lezak, 1992) is the Halstead–Reitan Battery (9 to 14 years) and the Reitan–Indiana Battery (5 to 9 years). The battery provides assessment of the broad domains of motor, visual–spatial, sensory–perceptual, attention, immediate memory, and abstract reasoning. Reitan and Wolfson (1985a) recommend that neuropsychological batteries include items that comprehensively evaluate brain functioning and strategies for interpretation of the findings, and that the procedures used have demonstrated empirical and clinical applications. Table 5.2 lists the measures included in the Halstead batteries.

Motor

Finger Tapping is a measure of motor speed and coordination. This test requires the child to tap a key as quickly as possible with first the index finger of the dominant hand and then the index finger of the nondominant hand. It is expected that the dominant hand will be faster than the nondominant. Grip Strength requires the child to squeeze as hard as possible on a dynamometer. Again, it is expected that the dominant hand will be stronger than the nondominant. Both of these measures test the motor cortex of the frontal lobe. The Tactual Performance Test requires the child to place forms into a form board while blindfolded, first with the dominant and then with the nondominant hand. This test yields three measures: Time, Memory, and Localization. The Time measure is also believed to be a measure of the frontal lobe, particularly the motor cortex. The Marching Test, for younger children, requires the child to touch a series of circles as quickly as possible using the dominant, nondominant, and both hands together. This measure is believed to be a measure of fine motor function and coordination.

Visual–Spatial

Trails, Part A, requires the child to connect numbers as quickly as possible. In the younger child's battery, Matching Figures, V's, and Pictures require the child to match figures and pictures as quickly as possible. The concentric square requires the child to copy the square. The Target Test requires the child to tap a series of dots after a short delay as modeled by the examiner. These measures are believed to tap visual–perceptual and motor skills

TABLE 5.2. Halstead Batteries

Domain	Halstead–Reitan (9–14 years)	Reitan–Indiana (5–9 years)

Motor	Finger Tapping
	Grip Strength
	Tactual Performance Test
	  (time)
		Finger Tapping
		Grip Strength
		Tactual Performance Test
		  (total time)
		Marching Test

Visual–spatial	Trails, Part A
	WISC-III subtests (Picture
	  Arrangement, Block
	  Design, Object Assembly)
		Matching Figures, V's, Pictures
		Target Test
		Concentric Square

Sensory–perceptual	Tactile Perception Tactile Form Recognition Tactile Localization Fingertip Writing Auditory Perception Visual Perception	Tactile Perception Tactile Form Recognition Tactile Localization Fingertip Writing
Attention	Speech Sound Perception Test Rhythm Test	Progressive Figures

Immediate memory	Tactual Performance Test—
	  Memory
	Tactual Performance Test—
	  Localization
		Tactual Performance Test—
		  Memory
		Tactual Performance Test—
		  Localization

Abstract reasoning	Category Test Trails, Part B	Category Test Color Form Test

most likely localized in the association areas of the brain (occipital, temporal, and parietal juncture).

Sensory–Perceptual

The Tactile Perception measure requires the child to interpret information provided through the fingers. The examiner touches the back of the child's hands separately or together, while the child's eyes are closed, for the Tactile Perception test. For Tactile Form Recognition, the child is asked to name objects placed in his/her hand while they are hidden and then to point to the figure identified through touch. The Tactile Localization test asks the child to identify the finger that is touched while his/her eyes are closed. For the Fingertip Writing task, X's and O's for the younger child and numbers for the older child are traced on the fingertips, and the child is asked to identify them. These measures evaluate parietal lobe functioning and the peripheral nervous system. All of these measures, however, can be confounded by poor attention and/or motivation.

The Auditory Perception Test requires the examiner to stand behind the child and move his/her fingers together by the child's ear (temporal lobe). For the Visual Perception Test the child's field of vision is checked through movement of the examiner's finger to the far left and far right in various positions (occipital lobe). These tasks can also be affected by poor attention and/or motivation.

Attention

The Speech Sound Perception Test requires the child to select the correct word as he/she hears it from a group of four. This task requires attention, but is also sensitive to difficulties in auditory discrimination and the ability to decipher words based on what is heard. This test can be negatively affected by reading difficulties and short-term memory deficits. The Rhythm Test requires the child to listen to 30 pairs of rhythm patterns and to tell whether the pairs are the same or different. This test is believed to measure auditory perception as well as concentration and attention. Progressive Figures, for younger children, requires the child to view an array of figures with smaller figures inside. The child must find the small shape, inside a larger figure, that is also on the outside. This test requires visual perception, speed, and attention.

Abstract Reasoning

The Category Test requires the child to determine a rule for a series of problems. The rules stay the same through each section but can change at the end of each section. In addition, the final segment requires memory of previously solved problems. This test requires problem-solving skills, memory, and cognitive flexibility as well as learning skills. Trails, Part B, requires the child to connect numbers and letters in alternating order as quickly as possible. This test is a measure of working memory. Both of these measures are believed to be sensitive to global functioning. The Color Form Test, for younger children, requires the child to touch figures in an order progressing from shape to color to shape, and so on.

Interpretation

The Halstead batteries can be interpreted using different approaches, including level of performance, pattern of performance, right–left differences, and the pathognomonic sign approach. Level of performance evaluates the degree to which the child is below average for his/her age, with two standard deviations being considered a significant deficit. Teeter and Semrud-Clikeman (1997) suggest that this approach be used only in conjunction with the other approaches because of problems with attention, motivation, psychopathology, or language deficits. Pattern of performance interpretation evaluates the child's strengths and weaknesses on the tests and makes inferences as to brain functioning based on this analysis. Evaluation of right–left differences requires the examiner to evaluate the child's performance on the tests that require handedness. Assumptions are made as to right or left hemispheric involvement particularly in the motor cortex. The pathognomonic sign approach requires analysis of certain items that are generally failed by people with brain damage. False negatives have been found with this approach, particularly in children who show wide variation in development that is still within normal limits (Teeter, 1986).

Interpretation of the Halstead batteries requires extensive training and supervision and should not be attempted by practitioners without such a degree of learning. Many neuropsychological reports may provide scores on the Halstead battery, and it is helpful for school personnel to understand what the tests are and what they measure.

The Halstead batteries have been well researched as to the utility of their measures. Intelligence has been found to be correlated with the Halstead batteries (Shurtleff et al., 1988) and may be responsible for the variation seen on the subtests, rather than the ability of the battery to discriminate between groups with special needs (Hynd, 1992). The battery has also been found unable to readily discriminate between psychiatric and brain damaged populations, as both groups perform poorly on these batteries (Hynd & Semrud-Clikeman, 1990; Tramontana et al., 1988). The batteries are time-consuming and expensive, with administration requiring 6 to 12 hours per client. Thus, the Halstead batteries can provide important information but require extensive training, expense, and time for administration.

Luria–Nebraska Neuropsychological Battery for Children—Revised

Interpretation of the Luria–Nebraska Neuropsychological Battery for Children—Revised (LNNB-CR) also requires extensive training and is presented here to provide an overview of the battery, not as a training exercise. The LNNB-CR is based on Lurian theory (1980) that describes brain activity as functional systems or units, as discussed in more detail in Chapter 2. The LNNB-CR (Golden, 1989) is developmentally based, in that skills are assessed according to what would be expected of a child at a certain age. There are 11 subtests of the LNNB-CR: Motor, Rhythm, Tactile, Visual, Receptive Speech, Expressive Language, Writing, Reading, Arithmetic, Memory, and Intelligence. Table 5.3 includes the measures in each section. Higher scores indicate poorer performance.

TABLE 5.3. LNNB-CR Subtests

Subtest	Areas measured
Motor	34 items measuring motor coordination, motor speed, and ability to copy geometric designs. Thought to measure motor cortex deficits.
Rhythm	8 items measuring perception, discrimination, and ability to reproduce rhythmic patterns. Measures of auditory perception and motor skills. Related possibly to right or left frontal lesions.
Tactile	16 items measuring the child's abilities on the right and left sides. Elevated scores related to parietal or parietal–occipital region deficits.
Visual	Child is asked to identify pictures, recall and draw figures, match and discriminate visual information. Elevated scores related to right posterior parietal–occipital regions or right anterior parietal when there are problems only in visual discrimination.
Receptive Speech	Child discriminates phonemes, reads words, is asked to comprehend words and sentences and to follow directions. Left hemispheric impairment implicated in higher scores.
Expressive Language	Child repeats simple and complex phrases, describes pictures, and discusses a picture or a short story. Generally sensitive to left hemispheric impairment.
Writing	Measures the child's ability to write, spell, and copy letters and words. Temporal–occipital–parietal juncture (angular gyrus) believed implicated in these tasks.
Reading	Child reads and listens to passages. Posterior association areas of the left hemisphere implicated in poor performance on this test.
Arithmetic	Requires the child to perform calculations (addition, subtraction, multiplication, division), recognize numbers, and complete story problems. Thought to implicate posterior left hemispheric regions.
Memory	Requires both verbal and nonverbal skills as well as short-term memory skills on tasks with and without cues. Appears to be most sensitive to verbal deficits.
Intelligence	Measures similar to the WISC are used, including similarities, vocabulary, comprehension, picture arrangement, picture completion, and arithmetic.

Interpretation

Qualitative as well as quantitative skills are required for interpretation of
LNNB-CR results. Determination of the presence or absence of brain damage through neurological evaluation and/or neuroradiological procedures is
important. Describing the child's strengths and weaknesses is a goal of this
evaluation, as well as determining the underlying causes of the behaviors

observed. Moreover, the LNNB-CR provides a method for determining a critical level of performance that differentiates brain injury from noninjury. This approach seeks to determine how many scales are above (poorer performance) or below a cutoff for the child's age level. When three or more scales are above this level, brain damage is a distinct possibility, whereas one or no scales above this level indicates normal functioning (Teeter & Semrud-Clikeman, 1997).

Research indicates that the LNNB-CR should be used with caution. It has been found useful in discriminating learning-disabled from nondisabled children (Lewis et al., 1993; Teeter et al., 1986) but not in identifying ADHD (Hynd, 1992; Karras et al., 1987). The usefulness of the battery for genetic and neurologically based disorders has not been fully established, nor its ability to correlate subtests with known lesions (Teeter et al., 1986). Thus, the LNNB-CR is not frequently utilized for neuropsychological evaluations and interpretation, and this battery should be used with caution.

Boston Process Approach

The Boston Process Approach does not utilize a battery of tests but is rather a hypothesis-testing approach, sampling specific behaviors such as memory, language, visual–motor, attention, reasoning, working memory, and perceptual–spatial skills. The approach requires the examiner to evaluate skills, progressing from the general to the specific, when less than optimal performance is seen. Thus, this method is not a published approach but varies according to the clinician and the client being seen. For this reason the examiner must be fully aware of a variety of measures and knowledgeable about performance at various developmental levels. Both qualitative and quantitative analysis are important in this approach, with a focus on using the results to develop an appropriate remediation plan (Milberg et al., 1986).

An interview generally begins the assessment, providing information about the child's history, premorbid functioning, levels of development, and current level of functioning. The emphasis is on the performance of the child and the testing of limits—evaluating how the child solves a problem. By sampling the child's ability through altering the task requirements, it is possible to determine whether the child's difficulty lies in retrieval, memory, time to complete a task, or poor strategies for learning. Kaplan (1988) proposes this approach as a way of gaining insight into brain–behavior functioning.

The strength of the Boston Process Approach is that there are no set tests required for administration, but an emphasis on skills and how the child solves problems. Yet this very strength is also the weakness of this approach, as it requires the examiner to be very familiar with a multitude of measures and to have sufficient experience and knowledge to apply observations to brain–behavior relationships. Further research is needed to determine the benefit of this approach for children and to provide the appropriate training in its use for the evaluation of children's needs.

TESTS FOR SCHOOL USE

Many tests can be employed by school psychologists to evaluate a child's learning and processing ability that are well within their training. A number of frequently used tests are listed in Table 5.4. This is not an exhaustive list, and additional measures are available in the field. It is intended to provide a guide for the school psychologist and related professionals (occupational therapists, physical therapists, speech pathologists) in conducting an assessment. These tests and their appropriate uses are discussed throughout this section. The publishers of selected tests are listed in the Appendix.

Cognitive and Academic Skills

IQ testing is one of the most common evaluations provided by school psychologists. Children with TBI may not show overall cognitive deficits after 6 months to 1 year of recovery based on an intelligence measure. This performance may not be sensitive enough to uncover learning difficulties, however, and further assessment is generally warranted. For other children with TBI, common measures of intelligence may not be appropriate, particularly when a child shows motor or attentional difficulties. Many suggest that IQ tests are too narrow to provide the information required for developing programs for children with TBI (D'Amato & Rothlisberg, 1996).

Verbal skills as measured by traditional IQ tests have been found to be fairly stable in children with TBI, and these tests may indicate higher levels of skills than are actually observed in the classroom and home environment (Ewing-Cobbs et al., 1986). Ylvisaker and colleagues (1990) suggest that the very standardized procedures used in the administration of these tests may inflate the scores. The one-to-one situation that decreases distractions and provides structure to the examinee may result in higher-than-expected scores, as may the examiner's ability to provide clear instructions and examples. In addition, the testing of skills across minutes (the usual delay is 20 to 30 minutes in length) rather than days may not be ecologically valid. Finally, the measurement of overlearned skills but not of newly acquired skills may indicate the possibility of a higher level of recovery than is actually present.

The WISC-III is the most commonly used measure of intelligence by clinical child and school psychologists (Sattler, 1990). Although it provides an excellent measure of intellectual functioning for children without head

TABLE 5.4. Suggested Psychological Measures for TBI

Test	Ages	Special considerations
Cognitive		
Wechsler Intelligence Scale for Children—III (WISC-III)	6 to 16-11	May not reflect child's functioning on different dimensions (working memory, executive functions). May penalize children with motor difficulty or difficulty with timing. Time required to administer may affect test scores.
Differential Abilities Scale (DAS)	2-6 to 17-11	Use of alternate procedures should be considered for children with motor and attention problems. Difficulty with motor control may lower scores on some of the subtests. Provides a comparison for visual and auditory short-term memory.
Kaufman Assessment Battery for Children (K-ABC)	2-6 to 12-11	Generally a nonverbal test; may be best for children with language difficulties. Motor components may be problematic for children with motor difficulties. Contains achievement subtests—some are culturally loaded and out-of-date.
Stanford–Binet Intelligence Scale—Fourth Edition (SB-FE)	2-6 to 23	May be appropriate for younger children. This test may not be useful for all children with language difficulties, as it requires abstract language skills on several subtests.
Achievement		
Wechsler Individual Achievement Test—II (WIAT-II)	6 to 17-11	Provides an overall score of a child's reading, mathematics, and written language skills. It does not provide enough "floor" to evaluate younger children's reading readiness skills. Attentional components may interfere with other children's performance.
Woodcock–Johnson Achievement Battery—III (WJ-III)	5 to adult	Concerns are similar to those regarding the WIAT-II. Use of the Word Attack subtest provides information as to the child's ability to decode words.
Kaufman Tests of Educational Achievement (KTEA)	5 to 18	Similar to the WIAT-II and WJ-III. This test is distinctive, as it provides a list of the child's academic strengths and weaknesses in various subcategories.
Peabody Individual Achievement Test—Revised (PIAT-R)	5 to 18	Similar to the WIAT-II and WJ-III.

TABLE 5.4. (*continued*)

Gray Oral Reading Test/Gray Oral Reading Test—Diagnostic (GORT and GORT-D)	6 to 18	Provide information as to the child's ability to read passages aloud as well as reading rate. Useful addition to the WJ-III or WIAT-II.
Memory		
California Verbal Learning Test— Children's Version (CVLT-C)	6 to 18	Child is required to learn a list of words with five repetitions. Provides measures of short-term and long-term memory. In addition, allows for the evaluation of the child's learning over time and ability to recognize information rather than just recall. Also allows for the evaluation of the child's learning strategies.
Wide Range Assessment of Memory and Learning (WRAML) and Test of Memory and Learning (TOMAL)	6 to 18	Provide information as to the child's ability to remember oral and visual information. The test may be confounded by attentional difficulties, and results may reflect such problems rather than memory difficulties. These tests are also very long, and the psychologist may wish to use certain subtests to evaluate the child's ability to learn (e.g., word–symbol, concentration tasks).
Children's Memory Scale (CMS)	5 to 16	Allows for evaluation of the child's memory and attentional skills. Provides various measures of visual versus verbal memory and short-term versus long-term memory. Good measure of the child's ability to recall information that is presented orally as compared with that presented visually. Also provides a separate scale to parcel out attentional effects on performance. This is a fairly new measure, and research is continuing on the uses of this test.
Executive functions		
Wisconsin Card Sorting Test	6 to adult	The child is required to match one of four cards by shape, color, or number. After 10 correct trials the rule is changed without the child's foreknowledge. Allows for evaluation of the child's problem-solving skills and ability to shift strategies. Can be a very frustrating task for some children and can provide a picture of their ability to deal with frustration. Scoring can be difficult, and additional training and supervision are required for use of this test.

(*continued*)

TABLE 5.4. (*continued*)

Stroop Color Word Test	7 to adult	Evaluates the child's ability to read words and identify colors and then to state the color of a word rather than the word itself (e.g., the word *red* printed in green). The test measures automaticity of overlearned skills and the ability to inhibit such skills. Norms are experimental, and the performance behavior of the child on this test may be more informative than the actual scores.
Category Test for Children	9 to 16	Part of the Halstead–Reitan Battery. Provides a measure of the child's problem-solving skills and includes a section on memory.
Verbal Fluency	9 to adult	Requires the child to name as many words as possible beginning with three letters: *f, a,* and *s.* It is a measure of the child's ability to retrieve information quickly.
Attention		
d2 Test of Attention	9 to adult	Requires the child to find targets within an array. Provides a measure of sustained attention, accuracy, and concentration. Easy to administer and score.
Gordon Diagnostic System, Test of Variables of Attention, Connors	5 to 17	Computer tests that measure the child's ability to attend to a target and ignore distractions within a time frame. Sensitive to attentional difficulties but also affected by processing problems. Even with significant attentional problems, older children and those with higher IQs may perform well on this task.
Language		
Clinical Evaluation of Language Fundamentals—3 (CELF-3)	6 to 21	Provides information as to receptive and expressive language. May be useful in evaluating more subtle language deficits and the child's ability to utilize language cues.
Peabody Picture Vocabulary Test—III (PPVT-III)	6 to adult	Provides a quick measure of receptive language skills. May be confounded by attentional difficulties.
Token Test for Children	4 to 12	Good measure of the ability to follow increasingly complex directions. Can be confounded by attentional difficulties.

TABLE 5.4. (*continued*)

Test of Language Development—3 (TOLD-3); 2 versions	4 to 8-11, 8 to 12-11	Provides measures of receptive and expressive language. Good visual cues provided.

Visual–motor

Bender–Gestalt	4 to 12	Good measure of visual–motor skills, but has limited norms past the age of 12. Also allows for a qualitative evaluation of the child's ability to organize visual information.
Beery Developmental Test of Visual–Motor Integration (VMI)	2 to 18	Provides a measure of the child's ability to copy increasingly complex geometric figures in a structured format. Allows for evaluation of visual discrimination and motor control.
Rey–Osterrieth Complex Figure Test	6 to adult	Requires additional training for scoring and interpretation. Provides information as to the child's visual–motor skills and planning and organizational abilities.
Motor–Free Visual Perception Test	6 to 12	Measures the child's ability to match figures based on orientation.
Judgment of Line Orientation	6 to adult	Provides information as to ability to understand spatial relationships. Is a nonmotor task, as child only needs to point to answer.

Motor

Purdue Pegboard	4 to adult	Provides information as to the child's ability to place pegs as quickly as possible with either hand and then with both hands together.
Grip Strength Test	6 to adult	Part of the Halstead–Reitan Battery. Provides measures as to hand strength. Requires additional training for interpretation.
Finger Tapping Test	6 to adult	Part of the Halstead–Reitan Battery. Provides measures comparing the two hands. Requires additional training for administration and interpretation.

(*continued*)

TABLE 5.4. (*continued*)

Neuropsychological

NEPSY	3 to 12	Provides information as to the child's language, attention, memory, visual–spatial, and visual–motor functioning. Various subtests evaluate the child's ability to process information both visually and verbally. Also provides qualitative measures of behavior. Requires a substantial background in neuropsychology for appropriate interpretation. Empirical support beyond the standardization is limited because of the newness of this measure.
Wechsler Intelligence Scale for Children— 3rd edition Process Instrument (WISC-III PI)	6 to 16	A newly published instrument that views the WISC-III through a neuropsychological lens and allows for interpretation of the processes underlying performance on the various subtests. This interpretative measure is promising in its use and may assist a professional with a background in neuropsychology to use the WISC-III in a more comprehensive and qualitative manner.

Behavioral

Rating scales, including the Behavior Assessment System for Children (BASC), Connors Behavior Rating Scales, Achenbach Child Behavior Checklist (CBCL)	2 to 18	All of these scales are well standardized and helpful. The BASC and the CBCL provide forms for the parent, teacher, and child.

injury, it may not be the best measure for children with TBI because of the reliance on speed and motor coordination for the performance subtests. In addition, it measures previously learned material but provides no index for material that is newly learned. Thus, the WISC-III can be helpful in evaluating the level of the child's previous learning but should not be used to measure the child's current learning skills. Studies have found that the WISC-III is most appropriately used to generate hypotheses rather than to measure intellectual potential (traditional use) for children with head injuries (Johnson, 1992).

There are similar concerns in regard to the DAS, although the timed tests can be administered using an alternate method. However, the DAS also relies on motor control for many of the spatial tasks, which may lower scores for children with motor difficulties. For example, a child that experienced a left-hemispheric stroke was evaluated in our clinic. He had previously been right-handed but now had right-sided hemiplegia. The Recall of Designs subtest of the DAS required control of a pencil to draw the figures; he experienced difficulty trying to draw the figures with his left (or nondominant hand). The K-ABC may be helpful for children with language difficulties. However, the motor components required in the hand movements subtest make it difficult for children with both motor and language impairment.

Cognitive tests should be used to provide a marker as to the child's verbal skills and previous learning. Interpretation of the performance subtests may be more difficult, and further evaluation is generally warranted. For children without TBI, IQ tests may be used to predict future performance. Such use of IQ tests for children with TBI is not appropriate. For these children, the IQ tests can provide information as to the current level of functioning but are not necessarily predictive of later functioning. These findings should be interpreted for parents and teachers in such a light, and serial evaluations are strongly recommended. In the first 5 years following injury, improvement has been noted in children with TBI (Semrud-Clikeman, 1999). Thus, during this period of time the child should be evaluated at least every 2 years if not every year. It is also very helpful to compare the raw scores on the subtests *as well as* the scaled scores. These comparisons enable the psychologist to determine progress in specific areas. On the verbal subtests, subtest scaled scores may show a slow decline that is due to a lack of new learning, not to a loss of skills. Comparison of the raw scores is important to determine whether no new learning is occurring or a true regression is in progress. Studies of the stability of IQ after TBI have found differential effects, depending on the location of the injury as well as the age of the child at injury. Children with damage prior to or during infancy have been found to show the lowest IQs, with lesion size being positively correlated to lower IQ (Banich et al., 1990). For children with left-hemispheric damage, the WISC results have been found to be fairly stable. Conversely, those with right-hemispheric damage show decreases on verbal IQ (VIQ), performance IQ (PIQ), and full scale IQ (FSIQ) over time (Aram & Eisele, 1994).

Academic assessment suffers from similar concerns as cognitive assessment. It is important to determine where the child started as well as any new learning that is occurring. Comparison of raw scores across administrations is also helpful in gauging the extent of new learning and enabling the psychologist to rule out a regression of skills. Elementary children have possibly learned sight words and word attack skills. But at fourth grade it may be reported that the development of reading comprehension and inferential thinking skills is not progressing as might be expected. As discussed earlier, it is possible that a child will grow into a deficit as he/she develops (Teeter & Semrud-Clikeman, 1997). A child who sustains TBI at age 5 prior to learning to read may develop reading difficulties in first grade that could not be evaluated at the time of the injury. The following case example illustrates this concern.

Josie was 4 years old at the time she climbed a tree and fell approximately 10 feet to a concrete patio at a babysitter's house. She experienced a left temporal hematoma and fractured skull, which required neurosurgery and removal of tissue in the temporal lobe. Prior to the accident Josie was described as good-natured, easy to discipline, having good attention for a 4-year-old and socially appropriate behavior. Josie was evaluated by a neurologist following recovery from surgery and found to be functioning well. A neuropsychological evaluation was not requested at that time. Her mother requested a psychological evaluation from the school system to determine whether Josie had any special education needs. The school psychologist administered the SB-FE and reported low average ability with no areas of weakness.

Readiness evaluation showed that Josie knew most uppercase letters and approximately half of the lowercase letters. She also knew the majority of colors, numbers, and shapes. No areas of concern were identified by this evaluation, and Josie was not considered for special education needs.

When Josie was 6 years old, her mother became concerned by her lack of progress in reading and number readiness, behavioral difficulties, which had not been present prior to the injury, and difficulty with attention. Family problems developed, as Josie's mother had become depressed, blaming herself and thinking that if she had not been working, Josie would not have fallen from the tree. Josie's father believed that his wife was overdramatizing the difficulty and that Josie was fine. According to her mother, Josie seemed more labile and easily frustrated. At times she was "in another world" and did not pay attention when people were talking to her. Particularly frightening to her mother was an occasion when Josie did not seem to recognize her uncle, who lived with the family. Josie's pediatrician conducted an EEG to rule out a seizure disorder, and the findings were reported to be normal. A neuropsychological evaluation was requested by the pediatrician to determine Josie's skills as well as her prognosis. The SB-FE was readministered to compare the scores from the previous evaluation. Both sets of scores are presented in the following chart, with results of the first administration shown in parentheses. A reminder: The average range for subtest scores is 42 to 58 and for composites, 86 to 116.

	Scaled score	Composite score
Vocabulary	40 (42)	
Comprehension	40 (48)	
Absurdities	38 (42)	
Verbal Composite		80 (90)
Pattern Analysis	41 (45)	
Matrices	44 (50)	
Abstract/Visual Reasoning		83 (90)
Quantitative	36 (38)	
Quantitative Reasoning		72 (80)
Bead Memory	36 (32)	
Memory for Digits	35 (44)	
Memory for Sentences	36 (36)	
Short-Term Memory		72 (80)
Composite		72 (85)

As shown in these SB-FE results, Josie's scores had declined since the initial evaluation. A comparison of the raw scores indicated that she had shown little growth in Vocabulary and Comprehension or in Quantitative Reasoning. Her Bead Memory score improved, whereas her Memory for Sentences stayed the same from the previous testing. Achievement testing indicated that she showed readiness skills at the same level prior to the accident. Her ability to pair sounds and symbols was below expectations for her age, as was her sight word vocabulary. Behavior rating scales completed by her teacher and parents indicated significant concerns about attention, withdrawal, and social skills. Josie's tendency to "daydream" was also evident during the evaluation, and concern was again expressed as to the possibility of a seizure disorder. A repeat EEG with sleep deprivation indicated abnormal signals and was read as being consistent with a partial complex seizure disorder. Josie experienced difficulty with new learning. Her initial SB-FE indicated previously learned material was retained. However, as she began first grade and was expected to learn sound–symbol relationships, Josie experienced increasing difficulty. Her undiagnosed seizure disorder further complicated the issue. In addition, family cohesion was an area of concern, and the stresses in the family were pronounced. These factors exacerbated the emotional difficulties seen in Josie and her mother.

Memory and Learning

The ability to remember something requires attention to the task, storage, and retrieval of the information. Memory deficits constitute a common cognitive problem in children with TBI and must be evaluated at various points in time. Particular difficulty has been found in the area of delayed memory, for which a full evaluation is strongly recommended (Lord-Maes & Obrzut, 1996; Reid & Kelly, 1993). Attentional difficulties can impair memory, and sorting out these two components can be difficult. Following the gathering of developmental information, it is important to evaluate, through parent and teacher interviews, the ability of the child to recall information over time. In addition, it is important to ask questions concerning the consistency of such recall—does the child remember items from day to day? Further information can be gathered as to the child's ability to recall incidents in his/her life or to retell a story or describe a television program. Although improvement in verbal memory has been seen over time, memory deficits persist even when there is improvement in cognitive functioning (Jaffe et al., 1990).

Table 5.4 provides information about the memory tests most frequently used in the field. The CVLT-C provides a measure of the child's ability to learn a list of words. The child's initial encoding of the list can be compared with how many words are learned after five trials. It is also possible to evaluate the child's use of memory strategies (grouping the items by category) and whether recognition improves the child's memory skills. The Test of Memory and Learning (TOMAL), Children's Memory Scale (CMS), and Wide Range Assessment of Memory and Learning (WRAML) also include tests that involve learning a list. These tests are good measures of the child's ability to learn new items and can suggest strategies for helping the child learn more efficiently.

The assessment of the child's ability to learn material within a context should also be evaluated. The general strategy in this type of evaluation is to read the child a story and see how much of the story he/she recalls. The WRAML and TOMAL provide this type of assessment as well as a measure of how much the child can recall when prompted by questions. Comparing the ability to learn word lists (nonmeaningful memory) with the ability to recall information within a context (meaningful memory) can assist in developing appropriate intervention strategies. If a child is helped to learn by the use of context, it will be important to provide learning experiences that build on experience rather than on rote memory. For example, if a child has difficulty with nonmeaningful memory, it will be difficult for him/her to learn to read using sight words or phonics. Rather, the child may profit from a strategy that uses a language-experience or whole-language approach in addition to the usual drill in phonics and sight words.

Attention

The assessment of attention is an important aspect of any evaluation, but particularly for children with TBI. Classroom observation is crucial for this type of assessment, as many children who otherwise have difficulty are able to pay attention in a one-to-one situation that is relatively free from distractions. Observing the child during structured and unstructured activities can allow a comparison of the child's ability to stay on task with and without teacher direction. It is also important to determine whether the child's attention fluctuates depending on the task at hand or time of day. Observing how the child manages transitions can provide valuable information about the child's ability to shift attention across situations.

Structured assessment of attention can be somewhat problematic, as many of the instruments are not fully empirically validated. Continuous performance tests allow for the evaluation of the child's ability to sustain attention, inhibit responding, and ability to be consistent over time. Such measures are fairly expensive and require a computer to be administered. If these tests are used, the child's performance should be monitored by the examiner.

The NEPSY includes an auditory and visual attention subtest that may be helpful with younger children. The visual attention task requires the child to select a target from an array as quickly as possible. The auditory attention task requires the child to listen for a target sound among similar sounds and to place a token in a box when the target is heard. Both measures are of interest in testing attention and appear to have promise. Although the NEPSY is intended for children up to age 12, these measures are likely most appropriate for children in the middle ranges, as the ceiling may be too low for the brighter and older child.

The d2 Test of Attention requires the child to select a target from an array as quickly as possible. The child is presented with a page of 14 lines, with the targets interspersed among similar distractors. Each 20 seconds, the child is asked to move down a line. The test provides a measure of attention, as well as accuracy and concentration, and is appropriate for participants aged 9 to adult.

Memory versus Attention

At times it can be difficult to evaluate the contribution of attention difficulties to memory problems. For example, if something is not paid attention to, it is likely that it will not be remembered. Therefore, it is important to make sure the child's attention is focused before beginning a task. Observation of the child may assist in teasing out the contribution of each of these factors in an assessment. It can be helpful, before beginning the test, to prompt the child to pay attention. Such prompting can assist the memory component and may be helpful in determining the contribution of attentional deficits to the problem. At times, I administer two similar tasks on different days—in one instance asking the child to carefully pay attention, and in the other not providing such prompts. In this situation, the performances can be compared to determine any differences that emerge. The

CVLT-C can be used one day, and the list learning from the TOMAL or WRAML on the next, or vice versa.

It is important to determine the contributions of both factors, as remedial strategies can differ accordingly. Moreover, if attention and memory deficits co-occur, the difficulty may be more severe and require more specialized interventions. Evaluation of both areas is required to develop the most appropriate educational program.

Executive and Reasoning Skills

Measures of executive functioning seek to test the child's ability to solve problems as well as his/her cognitive flexibility. These skills are important for functioning in everyday life, and difficulty in this area may significantly affect the child's adjustment and psychosocial functioning. Such measures can also provide information about the child's ability to cope with frustration and the strategies he/she may use.

One of the main aspects of executive functioning is a person's ability to develop insight into his/her own weaknesses and strengths. When there is a deficit in this area, remediation of the target problems becomes much more difficult. In addition, psychosocial functioning can be negatively affected by problems in insight, as the child/adolescent does not learn from previous experience or may be unable to transfer learning to various situations. In conjunction with the development of insight is the ability to set attainable goals. It is important that an interview provide information about the child's ability not only to set goals but also to understand the steps leading to these goals. Integral to these skills is the child's ability to self-monitor his/her behavior and to correct or redirect behaviors that are not helpful. Cognitive flexibility is very important in this area, allowing the child to select or reject various problem-solving strategies.

One of the major instruments used for assessment of executive functions is the Wisconsin Card Sorting Test. This instrument measures the child's ability to shift a cognitive set and to use strategies. The test can be quite challenging to administer and is difficult to score without extensive training. For most school psychologists, this measure may not be feasible.

The Stroop Color Word Test may also be helpful as a measure of inhibition. This test has three major parts, in which the child reads color words, then identifies colors, and finally states the color of a word rather than the word itself. The final task is a measure of inhibition because it requires the child to state a color that competes with a word. For example, the word *red* is printed in green ink and the child must read "green." The norms for this test are experimental, and interpretation of the test must be done carefully and conservatively.

The NEPSY includes a measure of executive functioning, named the

Tower. This test is similar to a well-researched measure frequently used in neuropsychological assessment and research, named the Tower of London or the Tower of Hanoi. The test requires the child to plan a strategy to replicate placement of balls on pegs within a specified number of moves. As such, it requires planning and organization as well as working memory. Norms are provided for children from 6 to 12 years of age. Qualitatively, it can be quite helpful to ask the child how he/she solved the problems. Thus, it is possible to evaluate potential learning strategies and the child's ability to compensate for difficulties.

In addition to these tests, one can also utilize measures included in traditional IQ tests. The Matrices subtest of the DAS lends itself to evaluation of the child's ability to use reasoning skills. Moreover, the Concept Formation and Analysis–Synthesis subtests of the WJ-III can also be helpful in evaluating the child's ability to reason and solve problems. These tests can be combined to obtain a measure of fluid reasoning and to gain information about the child's ability to solve novel problems.

Further information can be obtained about the child's reasoning skills through an analysis of his/her performance on the reading comprehension subtests of the WIAT-II and KTEA. Children who experience difficulty with inferential reasoning may do poorly on those items that require a conclusion to be drawn from the information provided and those that rely on concepts underlying the passage. Children with moderate to severe TBI often have difficulty with this type of reasoning even while being adept at searching for factual information. Reports on these skills by the child's teacher can also be helpful. Finding the main idea of a text can be difficult for children with TBI. Such difficulty can interfere with performance in higher-level classes in literature and compromise the ability to draw conclusions from a text, thus leading to problems in general academic functioning. Interventions needed for the development of these skills are discussed in Chapter 8.

As discussed earlier, formal achievement testing may not be sensitive to a child's learning difficulties. The use of curriculum-based material appears to be most appropriate for evaluating the child's progress over time. The use of class materials, as well as probes into how the child has solved problems, can be very useful, particularly in evaluating the child's problem-solving skills. In addition, the use of classroom materials can be ecologically valid as a means of assessing teacher expectations and the child's facility with worksheets.

Visual–Motor and Perceptual Skills

Deficits in visual–motor and perceptual skills are seen in approximately one-third of children following TBI (Levin & Eisenberg, 1979). Copying geometric figures, constructing block designs, and facial discrimination are areas that frequently prove difficult and appear more affected than verbal skills (Jaffe et al., 1990). Speed in visual processing and visual–motor skills have been found to be very sensitive to TBI (Chadwick et al., 1981b). An assessment must evaluate functional academic skills, such as handwriting, providing adaptations as needed. In addition, an evaluation of the child's handwriting speed is also needed. Difficulties in the speed of visual–motor skills can be due to motor dyscoordination, poor visual and perceptual skills, and/or attentional difficulties (Ylvisaker et al., 1990). It is important to determine whether one or more of these variables is affecting the child's handwriting skills.

The most frequently used measures for assessment of a child's visual–motor skills are the Bender–Gestalt and the Developmental Test of Visual–Motor Integration (VMI). The Bender–Gestalt test requires the child to copy nine figures on a page. Organization and structure are loosely provided, and this test offers an opportunity to evaluate the child's ability to plan his/her drawings. Some children may use a whole page, run out of room, and then return and draw over the original drawing. Others may carefully plan how they will make a drawing fit on one page. Although this test is designed as a measure of visual–motor skill, the astute clinician can also use the test to evaluate planning and organization.

In contrast, the VMI provides a structured format in which each item is presented within a set grid. The test allows for no erasures, so behavioral observations of impulsive responding are important. At times it can be quite helpful to compare performances on the Bender–Gestalt and the VMI to determine whether structure improves performance. Interventions for difficulty in planning and organization differ from those for a visual–motor deficit, and such information is important. If impulsive responding and attentional deficits are hampering performance, the interventions would address these difficulties. Furthermore, it is important to evaluate the speed of performance—a carefully completed Bender–Gestalt or VMI test that requires substantially more time than would be expected may indicate difficulty with speed or some compulsivity.

In addition to the VMI, measures that utilize perceptual skills in the absence of motor ability may be helpful in deciphering a deficit. The Judgment of Line Orientation Test (JLO) requires the child to choose lines that are in the same orientation as those in a sample. Motor skills are not crucial to this test, but it can be confounded by lack of attention, and such observations are important. The Arrows subtest in the NEPSY provides similar information to the JLO and can be considered for use in screening these skills.

Motor measures generally include the Purdue Pegboard, Finger Tapping Test, and Grip Strength Test. The Finger Tapping Test and Grip Strength Test are part of the Halstead–Reitan batteries and require some additional training for correct interpretation. The Purdue Pegboard, however, is fairly straightforward and can be used by school psychologists and/or occupational therapists quite readily. It requires the child to place pegs within 30 seconds, first with the dominant hand and then with the nondominant hand. Finally, both hands are to be used simultaneously within 30 seconds. Norms are available for performance and can be transformed into z scores (number of pegs placed – number for age and sex/standard deviation for age and sex) for age and sex.

Psychosocial, Emotional, and Behavioral Functioning

Assessment in the area of psychosocial, emotional, and behavioral functioning is particularly important, not only to understand the child's current emotional state but also to evaluate the possible effects of cognitive deficits on his/her functioning level. It is important to include an interview of the child and parent that encourages sharing of information as to the child's feelings, peer relationships, and emotional well-being at various times during recovery (Semrud-Clikeman, 1995). Behavior rating scales can be quite helpful in evaluating the child's functioning level, and the Behavior Assessment Scale for Children and the Achenbach Child Behavior Checklist provide very good information, as gained from the teacher, parent, and child/adolescent. The BASC allows for comparison of the various informants for areas of agreement and disagreement. The Connors scales provide information about the child's behavior and attentional abilities and can be quite useful for this type of evaluation.

Self-report measures can be useful when the child shows some degree of self-awareness. Such measures, however, can be problematic when a child is invested in presenting him/herself as having no difficulties or when insight is lacking (Semrud-Clikeman et al., in press). Measures that are frequently utilized in the field include the Children's Depression Inventory (CDI; Kovacs, 1992) and the Revised Children's Manifest Anxiety Scale (RCMAS; Reynolds & Richmond, 1978). These scales provide a screening to determine whether a more formal assessment of depression should be conducted. Measures such as the Rorschach and the Thematic Apperception Test require extensive training and may not be feasible for many school personnel to complete. They can provide useful information about a child's feelings and ability to resolve difficulties. The Roberts Apperception Test has also been used to provide such information, and many school districts have employed this measure.

USE OF ASSESSMENT FOR HYPOTHESIS
TESTING AND INTERVENTION

In many evaluations it is appropriate to use test scores for prediction of the child's functioning in the future. However, for children with TBI tests should be used to serve a hypothesis-testing approach to determine the strengths and weaknesses of the child with an eye to appropriate educational placement and intervention. For children with TBI the initial assessment, generally conducted in a hospital or outpatient setting, provides an indication of the child's level of functioning after the accident. It is not until the child returns to the school that one can fully appreciate the extent of learning difficulties or evaluate the child's response to the environment. Thus, follow-up evaluations must be used to check on the progress of the child and to form hypotheses about the child's development and strengths and weaknesses. In evaluations of other children we generally seek to diagnose learning problems or emotional difficulties based on the test scores. For children with TBI it is important to view the tests as a way of organizing information on the child's progress and to provide a description of his/her skills so that the multidisciplinary team can form the most appropriate IEP and treatment plan (Ylvisaker et al., 1990). It is suggested that this process continue throughout implementation of the treatment plan.

For assessment to be instructive for remediation, it is important that it encompass three main dimensions. First, evaluation of the child's ability to complete work in a timely manner provides insight into the efficiency of the child's problem-solving skills as well as motor components that may interfere with functioning. Second, evaluation of the child's ability to complete both concrete and abstract tasks can indicate areas for intervention. A child who is able to locate factual information but experiences difficulty with abstract reasoning may function well in the elementary grades but experience significant problems in middle school and high school. Finally, evaluation of the behaviors the child shows during problem-solving tasks is important for developing the remediation plan. Impulsivity, disinhibition, flexibility of thought and behavior, degree of independence, motivation levels, and awareness of abilities are areas of importance for adaptive functioning (Ylvisaker et al., 1990).

In addition to the aforementioned dimensions, it is also imperative to evaluate the environment in which the child is placed. A teacher's understanding of the effects of TBI or other brain deficits can go a long way in assisting the child in his/her transition. Although TBI as a category is now a fundable designation, many children with TBI are placed with special education teachers who have knowledge about learning disabilities and/or emotional disturbances but not necessarily about TBI. Regular education teachers may have even less information about TBI and thus need additional support.

For example, Susan, a child who had been in a coma for 2 weeks following a head injury sustained in a car accident, was reintegrated into a regular second-grade classroom. She had experienced significant brain swelling that required neurosurgery, as well as left-sided impairment. Initial neuropsychological evaluation indicated relatively intact skills with some problems in memory and language. Susan's neurosurgeon had cleared her for a full day in school with restrictions only on contact sports and overexertion. Special education services were provided for memory and language as well as for the academic subjects of reading and writing. Mathematics skills appeared to have been spared. Susan's mother contacted the neuropsychologist and requested a school meeting because Susan's teachers were complaining that Susan was "lazy and unmotivated." The meeting was quite fruitful, as it quickly became evident that there was little understanding as to the mechanisms of Susan's difficulties and the extent of her injury. Because she generally was functioning well physically, her teachers had mistakenly interpreted such functioning as indicative of intact skills and few deficits. During the meeting it was discovered that Susan's motivation level appeared to drop after about 10:00 A.M., then pick up after lunch, only to sag again at about 2 P.M. The school day lasted from 8:30 A.M. to 3:30 P.M. Upon discussion, it became evident that Susan was showing fatigue as a result of the long school day and that a rest period, both in the morning and in the afternoon, would be in her best interest. She was also referred to her doctor to determine whether she was showing hypoglycemia, or low blood sugar. These tests were negative. Susan's schedule was adapted and her functioning improved. This example illustrates that knowledge of the behavioral characteristics frequently accompanying TBI can assist in the appropriate interpretation of the child's skills and lead to suitable interventions.

It is important for the school psychologist and other professionals (occupational and physical therapists, speech–language pathologists) to provide information to school personnel about the difficulty the child may experience. Inservices are particularly relevant for school personnel in this area. There is emerging evidence that children who have the cognitive skills to function appropriately may fail to do so, given a faulty environment as was found in the preceding example (Ylvisaker et al., 1990). Thus, to be most usable and interpretable, assessment results must answer questions posed by teachers and parents.

Children with TBI may show inconsistencies across situations and tasks, and such fluctuation can result in misinterpretation of their abilities (Cohen, 1986; Ylvisaker, 1986). Our ability to predict a child's eventual outcome is problematic, as many children with TBI have experienced learning and behavioral difficulties prior to their injuries. Children with TBI can show average or above average IQs and academic grade-level achievement, yet perform very poorly in the classroom (Klonoff et al., 1977). It is important to assist teachers and parents in understanding this complex picture and to refrain from making predictions about future functioning. Continued special services should be supported with ongoing assistance for the family and teaching staff.

CHAPTER 6

♦♦♦

Two Assessment Examples

♦

The following case studies are presented as examples of assessments used to provide services to a child with a severe head injury to another with a moderate head injury. Richard's case (Case 1) has been discussed throughout this text, and the results of his assessment are provided here.

CASE 1: RICHARD

Richard, a 16½-year-old male, was recovering from a head injury suffered when he hit a tree head-on with his car. He had been in a coma for 3 days following the accident, had been hospitalized for 2 weeks, and had been in a rehabilitation center for the past 3 months prior to his evaluation. His history indicated that he had been a strong honors student with many friends and extracurricular activities. He was being readmitted to his school following recovery. Test results and all relevant information were presented at a planning meeting concerning his reentry. Those in attendance included the following hospital personnel: the pediatric neuropsychologist, occupational therapist, rehabilitation teacher, and case manager (registered nurse on the rehabilitation unit). School personnel included the school psychologist, school nurse, special education director, special education teacher, and occupational therapist.

Background Information

Richard lives with his mother, father, and four brothers in a rural town. Up until the time of the accident Richard was reported to have shown good development with no areas of concern. Emergency room records following the incident indicated a Glasgow Coma Scale (GCS) score of 5, with concerns expressed as to a possible skull fracture in the frontal area. CT indicated a skull fracture in the frontal area with a hematoma present. Intracranial pressure was elevated but was reduced with the administration of medication. Richard was in a coma for 3 days and awakened with no apparent difficulty in language. Upon awakening, Richard complained of frontal headache, dizziness, and nausea. Subsequent neurological examinations revealed some difficulty with fine motor control, particularly with the right hand, and difficulty with balance. Memory difficulties were also noted, particularly in short-term memory for digits.

Developmental History

Richard was the result of a normal pregnancy and delivery and weighed 7 pounds 12 ounces at birth. He was reportedly normal and healthy at birth. All of his early milestones were reported to have occurred within normal limits. Richard was reported to have been a happy toddler and had no unusual or extreme behaviors. His mother also reported that his health has been good.

School History

No difficulties were reported in Richard's progress throughout school. He generally obtained A's and B's and was described as a motivated child and adolescent with no behavioral difficulties. Richard was reported to have several friends and to enjoy hunting and fishing.

School records indicate no areas of concern during his development. Standardized achievement testing indicated above average reading and language skills from the very beginning of second grade until the present time.

Medical History

Richard's mother reports that following the accident he experienced short- and long-term memory difficulties, which have improved over time. She also reports that he has had some loss of feeling in his hands, severe headaches accompanied by vomiting and stomachaches, disorientation, and balance problems. She also noted sleepwalking and restless sleep.

Previous Testing

A neuropsychological evaluation of Richard was completed prior to his discharge from the hospital and admission to the rehabilitation center. This evaluation revealed high average intellectual ability (full scale IQ = 111) on a prorated WISC-R. Verbal skills were at 116 with performance abilities at

100. A moderate impairment in mental flexibility were and mild difficulty in word retrieval, orienting to novel tasks, and memory found. Significant deficits were found in balance, gross motor skills, fine motor skills, and motor dexterity. The recommendation was for placement in a rehabilitation center, occupational and physical therapy, and a 6-month neuropsychological evaluation.

Richard was last seen by a pediatric neurologist shortly after his discharge from the rehabilitation center. This examination was for evaluation of multiple complaints following his head injury. These concerns included headaches in the right frontal region, which were described as pounding and occasionally associated with nausea and vomiting if severe. Neck pain was an additional area of concern. The neurological examination indicated no focal deficits. An EEG and MRI scan were ordered to rule out a central nervous system structural lesion, and a neuropsychological assessment was recommended. The MRI results indicated normal intracranial contents and benign sinus disease, particularly in the right maxillary sinus. Results of the EEG indicated a normal waking pattern with no epileptiform activity

Behavioral Observations

Richard was seen for 2 days for the assessment. He was accompanied by his mother to these sessions and was cooperative, friendly, and well focused through the evaluation. He reported that he did not have a headache on either of the testing occasions. Richard attempted all tasks and appeared to do his best to complete them. Richard's verbal skills were intact, his speech understandable, and his spontaneous conversation appropriate for his age. His affect was full and varied, and he was very pleasant and interactive. The following results are believed to be a valid and reliable index of Richard's current level of functioning.

Test Results and Interpretation

Tests Administered

The following tests were administered for Richard's assessment: Wechsler Intelligence Scale for Children—III (WISC-III), Test of Variables of Attention (TOVA), Wechsler Individual Achievement Test (WIAT), Wide Range Assessment of Memory and Learning (WRAML), Wisconsin Card Sorting Test (WCST), Trailmaking Tests A and B, Grooved Pegboard, Developmental Test of Visual–Motor Integration (VMI), Personality Inventory for Children—Revised (PIC-R), Behavior Assessment System for Children— Parent Version (BASC), Children's Depression Inventory (CDI), and Revised Children's Manifest Anxiety Scale (RCMAS), Clinical Interview.

Cognitive Functioning

The WISC-III was administered to provide a measure of Richard's overall intellectual abilities. The test is divided into two parts: a Verbal Scale and a Performance Scale. The Verbal Scale consists of subtests that assess word knowledge, verbal problem-solving skills, general information, verbal abstraction, and auditory memory. The Performance Scale includes tests used to measure nonverbal abstraction and problem-solving skills, visual–perceptual skills, and sequencing ability. The scores obtained on each of the scales can be compared with average scores of 100, with the broad average range defined as 85 to 115. Richard's performance on the WISC-III is summarized in the following table. It should be noted that scaled scores of 7 to 13 define the average range of ability.

Verbal IQ	122
Performance IQ	100
Full scale IQ	112

Information	13	Picture Completion	10
Similarities	17	Coding	6
Arithmetic	12	Picture Arrangement	10
Vocabulary	13	Block Design	14
Comprehension	13	Object Assembly	10
Digit Span	7	Symbol Search	10

Richard achieved a full scale IQ of 112, which places him in the average range of intellectual functioning, and at the 61st national percentile, which means that Richard scored higher than 61% of children his age. His verbal IQ of 122 (90th percentile) is in the superior range, and his performance IQ of 100 (50th percentile) is within the average range of intellectual ability. There is a significant difference between Richard's verbal and performance abilities. The verbal score is slightly higher than that obtained 6 months earlier during the routine neuropsychological assessment, and the performance IQ is consistent with previous evaluation.

Richard shows overall superior skills in verbal comprehension. Superior skills were found on a measure of concept development, and above average skills were found in arithmetic reasoning, general fund of information, and vocabulary development. A relative weakness was found in Richard's ability to repeat digits.

Richard showed good development on tasks measuring his ability to pay attention to environmental detail, to complete visual reasoning tasks, and to perceptually analyze block designs and complete puzzles. Relatively weaker skills were found on a measure of visual–motor speed and on a task requiring planning. Results of these two subtests were mildly below average.

Attentional Functioning

The TOVA is a computerized measure of visual sustained attention providing indices of sustained attention, impulsivity, response time, and variability of response. Average standard scores are between 85 and 115. Richard's scores were as follows:

Omission (Inattention)	30^a
Commission (Impulsivity)	106
Response Time	44^a
Variability	52^a

[a]Below age expectations.

Richard showed significant difficulty on the TOVA, indicating problems with sustained attention, response speed, and variability of response. His impulse control was in the average range for his age. He showed average anticipatory responses but was slow in response time, showed a variable pattern of responses, and was unable to sustain attention on this task.

Memory Functioning

WRAML is a measure that assesses the child's ability to recall information both verbally and visually presented. This test includes a screening form that evaluates the child's ability to notice changes in a picture, recall a visual design after a short interval, learn a list of unrelated words over several trials, and recall a story that is read to the child. Average standard scores are between 85 and 115, and average scaled scores are between 7 and 13. Richard's scores were as follows:

Picture Memory	12
Design Memory	7
Verbal Learning	6
Story Memory	12
Memory Screening Index	100 50th percentile
Delayed Recall Subtests	
Verbal Learning Recall	Bright average
Story Memory Recall	Bright average

Richard shows average overall short-term memory skills. Particular strength was found on a measure of his ability to recall visual information and information provided in story format. Average skills were found on measures of visual memory and memory for a list of words repeated over time. Richard showed excellent long-term memory for the stories and list of words he had previously learned. Although a comprehensive comparison with previous memory testing is not possible, as that testing employed a measure primarily used with adults, Richard showed better ability at this testing than at his previous testing in short-term memory for information both within context and in list form.

Academic Functioning

The WIAT is a measure of general academic functioning in the areas of reading, arithmetic, and writing. On the reading subtests the child is asked to read single words and to read a passage and answer questions about content. On the arithmetic subtests the child is asked to solve word problems as well as general calculation problems. The writing subtests require the child to spell words and then to write a story on a topic. Average standard scores are between 85 and 115. Richard's scores were as follows:

	Standard score	Percentile
Basic Reading	80	9
Reading Comprehension	96	39
Reading Composite	84	14
Mathematics Reasoning	109	73
Numerical Operations	81	10
Mathematics Composite	96	39
Spelling	95	37
Written Expression	95	37
Writing Composite	95	37

Richard achieved a reading composite score in the below-average range and 28 standard score points below his full scale IQ. A discrepancy of such magnitude indicates significant difficulties in this academic area. Richard's basic reading skills indicate significant weakness in his ability to read single words. He did not show strong knowledge of phonetic rules, particularly for vowels. Richard seemed to read the words based on a sight word memory of the configuration. His mistakes included reading *phonograph* as *paragraph*, *ajar* as *ajer*, *ideally* as *edeally*, *poise* as *pose*, and so forth. Richard's comprehension skills, which were stronger, were in the average range. He was able to use contextual clues to figure out words he did not know.

On tests of mathematical ability, Richard showed strong average skills in mathematics reasoning ability. This score is commensurate with his arithmetic score on the WISC-III. Richard's numerical operations ability is significantly below his reasoning skills. He experienced difficulty with his knowledge of basic multiplication facts and was confused as to the process required for division problems and fractions. Richard's ability in written expression is in the average range. He made several spelling errors, but his ability to organize his thoughts and put them down on paper was good.

Richard appears to have significant difficulties in basic reading skills. He prefers to use a sight word approach, and this strategy becomes more problematic as words become more complex. Richard has learned to compensate for this difficulty through the use of contextual clues, and his reading comprehension skills are well within the average range. Although his difficulty with basic reading is also present in his spelling ability, Richard shows age-appropriate ability to express himself in written form.

The results of Richard's achievement testing were considerably below what would be expected of an adolescent with a 3.75 grade point average prior to injury. Although improvement has been seen, according to Richard's rehabilitation teacher, there are deficits in his learning skills, which will negatively affect his adjustment in school without support.

Executive Functioning

The WCST is a measure of executive or frontal lobe functioning, including the ability to form concepts, generate an organizational strategy, and use examiner feedback to shift strategy to the changing demands of the task. Richard's performance is summarized as follows:

No. of Categories Completed	6	Average to above average
Perseverative Errors	121	Above average
Failure to Maintain Set	0	Average to above average

Richard performed at the average to above average level on this task, indicating strengths in cognitive flexibility, problem solving, and response to feedback. This area was a strength for Richard, and improvement has been seen since the previous neuropsychological evaluation. He was able to shift solutions, depending on examiner feedback, and showed no perseverative errors, which indicates that he has well-developed cognitive flexibility.

Trailmaking Tests A and B were also administered. Trailmaking A requires the child to connect numbers in order as quickly as possible without making a mistake. Trailmaking B requires the child to connect numbers and letters in alternating order as quickly as possible without making a mistake. Higher positive scores indicate longer times to complete the task. Scores are converted to z scores, with average scores falling between +1.00 and −1.00. Richard's scores were as follows:

Trailmaking A	−0.38
Trailmaking B	−0.75

On both of these measures Richard showed age-level skills. He made no errors on these tasks. He performed significantly better than on his previous assessment. Richard's performance on Trailmaking B is commensurate with his good performance on the WCST, which is also a measure of cognitive flexibility.

Motor Functioning

The Grooved Pegboard is a motor task that requires the child to place pegs into keys arranged on a board. The test provides measures of motor quickness as well as errors. Scores are converted to z scores, with average performance ranging between −1.0 and +1.0. High positive scores are not desirable. Richard used his right hand as the preferred hand on this task. His scores were as follows:

Dominant Hand Time	+1.75
Dominant Hand Errors	0.00 Average
Nondominant Hand Time	+0.50
Nondominant Hand Errors	0.00 Average

Difficulty was noted with Richard's use of his dominant hand. Although he was accurate in the placement of the pegs, the time required to complete the task was above expectations for his age. Qualitatively, he experienced difficulty handling the pegs and positioning them on the pegboard.

The VMI is a measure of the child's ability to copy increasingly complex figures. Richard achieved a score of 80 on this test, which places him in the below average range. Previous evaluations had found functioning to be below 70, so there has been improvement on this measure. When the figures became more complex, Richard was easily frustrated with them and had difficulty making his hand go where he wanted. He became angry, and it was increasingly difficult for him to complete this task.

Emotional Functioning

Richard's adjustment was assessed through responses to the Behavior Assessment System for Children, which yields information about perceived cognitive, emotional, familial, and interpersonal problems, as well as parental test-taking attitudes. Richard's mother served as informant. T scores are reported in the following table, with an average of 50 and an average range of 40 to 60. Lower scores are desirable for the clinical scales, and higher scores are desirable for the adaptive scales. Richard's scores are as follows:

	T score	Percentile
Hyperactivity	46	37
Aggression	42	21
Conduct Problems	39	6
Externalizing Problems	41	16
Anxiety	36	3
Depression	37	5
Somatization	58	83
Internalizing Problems	43	22
Atypicality	54	75
Withdrawal	47	1
Attention Problems	60+	14
Behavioral Symptoms Index	44	31
Social Skills	49	45
Leadership	46	36
Adaptive Skills Composite	47	39

According to the parental form of the BASC, no significant difficulties for Richard were noted at home. Both clinical and adaptive skills are within average expectations for Richard on the BASC. Richard's attentional skills constitute an area of relatively greater difficulty than his other areas of development.

Because of his relatively elevated attention scores on the BASC and Richard's poor performance on the TOVA, a clinical interview, adapted from a structured clinical interview, was conducted with his mother; it yielded no DSM-IV diagnoses. His mother did not indicate significant concern with Richard's attentional problems. She did substantiate his having difficulty with paying close attention to details and making careless mistakes on schoolwork. Richard also completed this interview, reporting that he had difficulty listening to instructions when he had a headache, that he disliked doing tasks that require sustained effort, that he could be easily distracted, and that he could be forgetful. He did not meet the diagnostic criteria for ADHD based on either his or his mother's report.

The CDI requires the child to select statements that are most descriptive of his/her feelings. Richard scored in the average range on this measure. He did indicate a mild concern that his schoolwork was not as good as before, that he was not sure things would work out for him, that he worried that bad things might happen to him, that it was hard for him to make up his mind, and that he did not always like to be around people. Upon questioning, Richard indicated that he had concerns about how he was doing in school and would like help in English. He also mentioned that his headaches were of concern to him.

The RCMAS a true–false test; the child reads various statements and determines whether they are true or false of him/her. Richard scored well within the average range on all scales.

Impressions and Recommendations

Richard is a 16½-year-old Caucasian male who experienced head trauma when his car hit a tree. He was in a coma for 3 days and has been in a rehabilitation center for the past 3 months. Progress has been reported by the center, but there is still concern as to Richard's academic skills, low frustration tolerance, and mild attentional difficulties. His mother indicated that Richard experienced headaches, short- and long-term memory loss, and dizziness following the accident. He has had repeated neurological examinations, the results of which have been normal, and medications have been prescribed for his headaches, which are believed to be vascular in origin. Richard's mother reported that his memory difficulties and headaches have been decreasing. Richard's school history indicates above average performance with no areas of concern.

Richard's neuropsychological functioning is generally within age expectations. He shows average overall cognitive ability, with superior strengths in verbal comprehension and perceptual organization. There is mild difficulty in visual–motor speed and planning ability. Richard shows significant strengths in cognitive flexibility, problem solving, and response to immediate feedback. Both visual and auditory memory skills appear to be intact. Memory for details is enhanced when details are provided within a context. However, difficulties in motor skills and balance continue. In addition, Richard's frustration at his difficulties likely interferes with his performance on tasks requiring sustained effort and attention.

On a computerized measure of visual attention, Richard experienced difficulty in sustained attention, response speed, and variability of responding. A behavioral rating scale indicated mild concern on his mother's part as to Richard's attentional abilities. A clinical interview with both Richard and his mother indicated that he did not meet DSM-IV criteria for a diagnosis of attention-deficit/hyperactivity disorder, but yielded indications of mild difficulty in attention that should be addressed through behavioral means. These attentional difficulties are reported to worsen when Richard experiences a headache.

Richard showed academic difficulty in his performance on measures of achievement and in his progress in classes at the rehabilitation center. His reading skills are variable, with basic reading skills showing mild to moderate delays compared to his intelligence, and reading comprehension to be within expectations for his age and ability level. However, these deficits do not significantly interfere with his ability to comprehend what he is reading, which is the more important concern. Similarly, Richard shows adequate ability in written expression, with spelling errors consistent with his deficit in basic reading skills. These reading skill delays, coupled with attentional constraints, may make it difficult for Richard to complete his work in a timely fashion. Additional structuring and modification of tasks is necessary for Richard to be successful.

Emotional assessment indicated no significant areas of concern. Richard does express concern about his headaches but believes that their severity has lessened greatly over the past 2 years. There may be difficulty in Richard's overall adjustment to his injury. He expressed denial of his problems throughout the assessment. Although behavior rating scales indicated no difficulty, observations of his behavior and emotions during frustrating tasks, as well as reports from the rehabilitation center, indicate that he is having trouble coping with the aftermath of his injury. Although his academic skills are not up to the level at which they were prior to the accident, some improvement is likely over the next few months. Richard's reaction to these difficulties is of most concern, and psychological counseling may be helpful to him, as well as education concerning recovery from TBI. In addition, parent support appears appropriate, as his parents admit to wanting to protect Richard. Given that his driving privileges have been revoked, issues of individuation are likely to be paramount and to cause friction in the home. Education on these issues is particularly important for the family to support Richard's efforts to manage his feelings of anger and denial and his need to be independent.

CASE 2: KIMBERLY

The following case illustrates concerns that are frequently presented for evaluation. This child had a history of learning and attentional problems prior to her accident. These difficulties appear to have been exacerbated following the injury and to contribute to difficulties in treatment and interventions. The history of this child, previous evaluations, and test results and interpretations are presented here.

Background Information

Kimberly, a 13-year-old female, was referred for a neuropsychological evaluation of her level of functioning following recovery from a severe motor vehicle accident in which she was a passenger. At the time of the accident Kimberly was age 11½ and in fifth grade. The car in which she was riding was hit head-on by a driver who crossed the median on a divided highway. Her mother was thrown from the car; she sustained significant injuries to her internal organs, but no brain injury. Kimberly, not wearing her seat belt, hit her head on the windshield of the car. She was unconscious but breathing spontaneously when emergency medical services arrived on the scene. At the emergency room of the hospital Kimberly was comatose at that time, and a score of 4 was reported on the Glasgow Coma Scale (GCS). She did not withdraw from pain and showed little response. X-rays indicated broken ribs, and a CT scan showed a right cerebral hematoma in the parietal lobe and a frontal lobe skull fracture. In addition, Kimberly suffered from lacerations in her liver; her other internal organs were intact. A repeat CT scan 2 hours later found additional hemorrhages present. CT was repeated 12 hours later, at which time no new hemorrhages were found and no significant changes were noted. Eye opening did not occur until 15 days later. At that time Kimberly could sustain alertness and could follow the neurologist's finger with her eyes. She was then transferred from the intensive care unit to the general pediatrics ward with a GCS score of 10. Kimberly remained hospitalized for 2 additional months, and full evaluations were conducted in the areas of neuropsychology and speech and language pathology, and for occupational therapy.

Speech and Language Evaluation

Six weeks after the accident Kimberly was able to use single words but not sentences. Her attention had increased from 10 to 15 seconds to 10 minutes. During the initial 6 weeks of recovery she showed a slow rate of speech with poor articulation and a monotone quality. Treatment focused on improving auditory comprehension, expressive language, and problem-solving strategies. Formal assessment indicated the presence of a language disorder with impaired auditory retention and attention. Weaknesses in language were reported to have been present prior to the accident, but it was thought that these weaknesses had been exacerbated. Word retrieval and organization/planning of thoughts were believed to be additional areas of weakness, with strengths present in confrontational naming and word fluency. These difficulties were found to have resolved approximately 7 months after her discharge from the hospital.

Occupational Therapy

The initial occupational therapy evaluation indicated high muscle tone on the left side. Kimberly's dominant hand was her left. Additional areas of concern included balance, memory, problem solving, and impulse control. Therapy continued during the hospitalization and was further recommended upon reentry into school. During her recovery Kimberly received daily occupational therapy (OT), which was decreased in frequency at discharge from the hospital. Following school reentry, Kimberly was provided OT one time a week for 30 minutes. Difficulties were found in handwriting and with fine motor coordination. Cursive writing was problematic and very slow. Kimberly was reported to show a very low frustration tolerance and impulsive behavior. At times she became explosive when confronted with tasks on which she felt unsure.

Physical Therapy

Kimberly had balance problems following the accident. During her hospitalization she received physical therapy (PT). A reevaluation approximately 6 months after her awakening from the coma found significant gross motor problems, including difficulty with walking and running. Recommendations were for continued physical therapy at one to two times a week, and an ankle brace was ordered to improve stability on the left side.

Previous Neuropsychological Evaluations

Kimberly had been evaluated by her school system prior to the accident. At that time she had a verbal IQ (VIQ) of 131 and a performance IQ (PIQ) of 89, with some difficulties in mathematics calculation but strong skills in mathematics reasoning and reading ability. Two months after the accident Kimberly was evaluated by the hospital neuropsychologist. Results at that time indicated average cognitive ability (VIQ 98) but poorer nonverbal processing skills (PIQ 68) as compared with previous assessments by the school. Reading, spelling, and arithmetic skills were found to be within the average range, with arithmetic skills being relatively weaker. Deficits were also found in sustained attention, based on observation, but overactivity and impulsivity were not seen. Although a formal measure was not applied, deficits in memory were observed. Problem-solving skills were mildly compromised, and disinhibited behavior was seen throughout the testing. Handwriting skills were found to be below average.

Kimberly was reevaluated by the same neuropsychologist 5 months later to determine the course of her recovery. At that time Kimberly was found to have a VIQ of 98 and a PIQ of 72 on the WISC-III. These scores continued to be significantly poorer than they were prior to the accident. Significant difficulty was found in information-processing speed and on tasks that required Kimberly to organize information both visually and orally. Achievement testing indicated intact reading skills, with below average performance on arithmetic calculation and reasoning. Executive functions and attentional skills were found to be minimally impaired at the second evaluation. Memory dysfunction was reported most predominantly for visual information. No concerns were raised about how Kimberly had adjusted to her head injury.

Neurological Examination

Kimberly was evaluated 5 months after the accident by a pediatric neurologist. At that time she was attending school half days and was reported to be performing well. She was continuing to show mild left-sided weakness. Recommendations included monitoring by the physical therapist and a full day of school. Some problems with attention were found, but stimulant medication was deferred at that time. The neurologist also believed that no further substantial improvement would be seen and that these deficits would be permanent.

Medical and Developmental History

Kimberly's development was generally normal with no areas of concern. She was somewhat late in her ability to sit alone but quickly learned how to crawl, and then to walk by 12 months of age. Speech development was early, and she was reported to have put two or three words together by the time she was 13 months old. As a toddler, Kimberly's mother reported, she seemed to be overactive and very distractible. Kimberly was also reported to have more temper tantrums than most children her age. Her mother further reported that she had always seemed "quite fearless" and very social. Kimberly's medical history was generally nonremarkable prior to the accident.

School History

Kimberly's school history indicated that her elementary years were generally quite successful until she began fifth grade, when she was referred for an evaluation of a possible attention-deficit/hyperactivity disorder (ADHD). ADHD was ruled out at that time, but Kimberly qualified for learning disability services. An additional concern expressed was that Kimberly's mood appeared to be generally sad and negative. Classroom observations found her to have adequate attention but difficulty with organization. Teacher behavioral ratings reported no significant concerns. A speech and language evaluation indicated receptive/expressive language skills to be well above age expectations. Occupational therapy assessment found that Kimberly's running speed, agility, and balance were slightly below age level, with significant problems in fine motor skills. Parent reports indicated continuing concern with fine and gross motor skills. Recommendations were for occupational therapy focusing on arm and hand control for fine motor tasks and computer options to be explored as an alternative to writing. A written language and mathematics learning disability was diagnosed, and services were prescribed for these difficulties.

Kimberly was reevaluated by the school psychologist 12 months after the accident. Testing at that time indicated that her VIQ was at 121, which was slightly lower than at the previous testing, and that her PIQ had declined 17 standard score points (from 89 to 72). Her verbal scores fell roughly within the same pattern shown previous to the accident, with the exception of one subtest. Results of this subtest, which measures social judgment and reasoning, had declined from the superior range to the high average range. Particular decrement was found on the performance measures, especially in visual motor speed, visual reasoning, and the ability to replicate a block design.

An IEP for Kimberly included recommendations for an aide to assist with math assignments, adjustment of assignments as necessary, promotion to eighth grade, speech and language therapy, and occupational therapy. Kimberly's classification was changed from learning disability to traumatic brain injury (TBI). She was mainstreamed in all classes and receives weekly OT, PT, and speech and language therapies.

Current School Concerns

Kimberly was referred by her school district for additional evaluation 18 months after the accident, at age 13. She was obtaining A's and B's on tests, but in her daily work and on her report cards was receiving C's and D's. Her special education and regular education teachers expressed concern that Kimberly was showing attentional difficulties and problems with impulse control. The pediatric neuropsychologist worked in conjunction with the school district to determine Kimberly's needs.

Current Parent Concerns

Kimberly's mother has reported concerns about Kimberly's memory, her ability to follow directions, and her ability to finish her work. Difficulties in these areas have seemed to have increased since the accident. Her mother has also reported that Kimberly is experiencing some difficulty falling asleep and frequently wakes up at night. When she laughs, she drools and cannot seem to catch her breath.

Behavioral Observations

Kimberly was seen for 1 day for the evaluation. She was accompanied by her mother to the testing session and readily separated. Kimberly was cooperative, friendly, and well focused throughout the assessment. She attempted all tasks and appeared to do her best to complete them. She was distracted by noises in the adjoining room or in the hall but could easily redirect her attention.

Kimberly's verbal skills were excellent, her speech understandable, and her spontaneous conversation appropriate for her age. Her affect was full and varied, and she was very pleasant and interactive. She showed good attention to task and was able to screen out distracting noises. She reported that she enjoyed doing things with other children and that she liked her neighborhood because there were lots of friends available.

During the testing Kimberly frequently reminded the evaluator that she was very smart. However, during the second session she asked the examiner whether something was wrong with her brain and whether she would need help for the rest of her life. At that point Kimberly was willing to talk about her feelings concerning the accident. Her affect was subdued and generally sad at that time, although she appeared realistic in her appraisal of her strengths and weaknesses.

Kimberly responded very well to praise and worked diligently even on tasks that were somewhat difficult for her. She had a great sense of humor and frequently smiled throughout the assessment. The results obtained were thought to be valid and reliable.

Test Results and Interpretation

Tests Administered

The tests administered included the Differential Abilities Scale (DAS), Wechsler Individual Achievement Test (WIAT), Test of Variables of Attention (TOVA), Woodcock–Johnson Cognitive Battery—Revised (WJ-R), Test of Memory and Learning (TOMAL), Grooved Pegboard, Bender–Gestalt test, Judgment of Line Orientation test (JLO), Wisconsin Card Sorting Test (WCST), Behavior Assessment System for Children (BASC)—parent, teacher, and child versions, Children's Depression Inventory (CDI), Revised Children's Manifest Anxiety Scale (RCMAS), Rorschach Inkblot Test, and Thematic Apperception Test (TAT), Clinical Interview.

Cognitive Functioning

The WISC-III had been administered several times, yielding various scores. On this test, the reliance on motor skills and speed was of concern in the evaluation of Kimberly's skills. Therefore, the DAS was selected to tease out the motor component from the perceptual deficits. The DAS consists of core and diagnostic tests of general cognitive ability and an academic section. The cognitive subtests assess the child's ability to understand and use language, complete puzzles and block designs, and interpret visual information. The diagnostic subtests evaluate the child's short- and long-term memory and speed of information processing. Average standard scores for the general cognitive index are between 85 and 115, with average *T* scores for the individual subtests between 40 and 60. Kimberly's scores were as follows:

	Standard score	Percentile
Verbal Cluster	146	99.9
Nonverbal Reasoning	98	45
Spatial	74	4
General Cognitive Ability	106	66

Core subtests	*T* score
Verbal subtests	
Word Definitions	82
Similarities	72
Spatial subtests	
Recall of Designs	29
Pattern Construction	41
Nonverbal reasoning subtests	
Matrices	44
Sequential and Quantitative Reasoning	54
Diagnostic subtests	
Recall of Digits	41
Recall of Objects—Immediate	46
Recall of Objects—Delayed	30
Speed of Information Processing	36

Kimberly achieved a general cognitive ability score of 106, which places her in the average range as compared with children her age, and at the 66th national percentile. She achieved a verbal score of 146, which is in the very superior range as compared with same-aged peers, and at the 99.9th percentile. Her nonverbal reasoning score of 98 is within the average range and at the 45th percentile, and her spatial score of 74 is at the 4th national percentile. There is a significant difference between Kimberly's verbal abilities and her nonverbal reasoning and spatial skills. Her spatial skills are poorly developed, and the test results were negatively affected by a particularly poor score on recall of designs. This task required Kimberly to view a design and then draw it from memory. Kimberly's nonverbal reasoning skills are in the average range and are roughly equivalent to those determined in previous testing using the WISC-III. Her verbal skills are significantly higher on the DAS than on the most current WISC-III but are consistent with the initial evaluation prior to the accident.

On the verbal subtests Kimberly showed an exceptionally well-developed ability to define words and to describe how three words were similar (syrup, candy, cake = sweet). Her nonverbal reasoning skills that required no motor skill involvement were in the average range for her age. When children show physical disabilities, it is not recommended that the performance subtests of the WISC-III be used to estimate the child's ability, inasmuch as many of these tasks are timed and require motor control. Therefore, given her performance on the DAS, Kimberly's nonverbal reasoning skills were found to be intact when the motor component was eliminated.

Kimberly shows significant weakness in her ability to recall designs, a finding that contributed to her below average score on spatial skills. Her ability to copy block designs was within the average range for her age when speed was not required, and her score was considerably above the previous block design score on the WISC-III conducted after the accident. Thus, Kimberly's nonverbal skills, with the exception of visual memory, are well within expectations for her age and her verbal ability is in the very superior range.

The diagnostic tests indicated age-appropriate short-term memory for digits and objects, and delayed memory for objects significantly below average for her age. Kimberly's speed of information processing was also below expectations for her age and consistent with her mother's report of her "slowness" in response.

Attentional Functioning

The TOVA is a computerized measure of visual sustained attention and provides indices of sustained attention, impulsivity, response time, and variability of response. The first half of the test presents the stimulus less frequently, and the second half presents the stimulus more frequently. Average standard scores are between 85 and 115. Kimberly's scores were as follows:

	Total	1st half	2nd half
Omission (Inattention)	76[a]	66[a]	82
Commission (Impulsivity)	96	99	96
Response Time	73[a]	47[a]	81
Variability	74[a]	69[a]	86

[a]Significantly below age expectations.

Kimberly shows scores in the below average range overall on the TOVA, indicating mild problems with sustained attention, response speed, and consistency of response. Her ability to inhibit responding is in the average range for her age. When her scores for the first and second halves of the test are compared, Kimberly shows improvement in the second half on all measures except Commission, which was in the average range throughout the test. Thus, when the task required more responses, Kimberly performed in the average to low average range.

Memory Functioning

The TOMAL is a measure that assesses the child's ability to recall information both verbally and visually presented. The TOMAL provides scores for tasks that require both short-term and delayed memory for verbal and nonverbal information. In addition, there are scales evaluating the child's ability to attend to a task, recall information that is provided in serial order, recall information without prompts, recall information that can be associated with other information, and show improvement in performance over time. Average standard scores are between 85 and 115, and average scaled scores are between 7 and 13. Kimberly's scores were as follows:

	Standard score
Verbal Memory Index	78
Nonverbal Memory Index	83
Composite Memory Index	80
Delayed Recall Index	82
Attention/Concentration Index	97
Sequential Recall Index	90
Free Recall Index	75
Associative Recall Index	88
Learning Index	77

Verbal subtests	Scaled score
Memory for Stories	10
Word Selective Reminding	7
Object Recall	3
Digits Forward	8
Paired Recall	6
Letters Forward	9
Digits Backward	4
Letters Backward	6

Nonverbal subtests	
Facial Memory	3
Visual Selective Reminding	10
Abstract Visual Memory	9
Visual Sequential Memory	6
Memory for Location	10
Manual Imitation	11

Delayed recall subtests	
Memory for Stories	8
Facial Memory	4
Word Selective Reminding	6
Visual Selective Reminding	11

Kimberly's performance on the subtests was variable and ranged on both verbal and nonverbal tasks from significantly below average to average. All of these scores are significantly below expectations for her verbal ability. On the verbal subtests Kimberly showed age-appropriate skills in her memory for stories, recalling a list of words, and ability to recall digits and letters. Her performance on a paired associative learning task and her ability to repeat letters and digits in reverse order were below average. The paired associative learning task requires the child to learn pairs of words, some of which are easily associated (up–down) and some of which are hard (cabbage–pen). Kimberly readily learned the easy associations, but for the harder ones gave related items, similar to those presented in the easy associations. Repetition of the correct response did not change Kimberly's answer. Significant weakness was found on a measure of her ability to recall objects that were serially presented to her in five trials in different orders. In contrast, Kimberly was able to recall objects on the DAS when they were presented in the same order.

On the nonverbal subtests Kimberly showed age-appropriate skills in her ability to recall patterns when presented over successive trials, to recall abstract designs presented over five trials, to recall locations of designs, and to imitate hand movements. Below-average performance was found on a measure that required her to recall pictures in order. She showed significant weakness on a test of facial memory.

Measures of delayed recall indicate that Kimberly showed age-level ability to recall three stories and a pattern after a 30-minute delay. Her performance was below average for memory of faces and for a list of words she had previously learned. The supplemental indices indicate that Kimberly showed age-appropriate performance on measures of concentration and attention, ability to recall information that was serially presented, and ability to associate information with a cue in order to recall it. Below average performance was found in her ability to recall information without prompts and in her ability to learn information over successive trials. On the learning trials, Kimberly improved her learning with each successive trial but not to the level achieved by most children her age. This finding was particularly evident in regard to visual information, whereas verbal information showed the normal progression expected of a child her age.

Thus, similar to previous assessment results, Kimberly showed delays in visual memory but her verbal memory was relatively intact. Her attention and concentration ability appears to be within average expectations on this measure. Particular difficulty was found in her memory for faces, a finding not uncommon in children with nonverbal learning disabilities.

Academic Functioning

The WIAT includes measures of word reading, reading comprehension, basic number skills, mathematics reasoning, spelling, and written expression.

On the reading subtests the child is asked to read single words and then to read a paragraph and answer a question about content; the basic number skills requires the child to complete calculation problems, with the reasoning task requiring the solution to word problems; the spelling subtest requires the spelling of common words; and the written expression subtest requires the child to write an essay on a selected topic. Average standard scores are between 85 and 115. Kimberly's scores were as follows:

	Standard score
Word Reading	123
Reading Comprehension	110
Mathematics Reasoning	100
Numerical Operations	77
Spelling	102
Written Expression	80

Kimberly achieved a score in the superior range on word-reading skills and had average reading comprehension. She showed good use of phonics as well as an excellent sight word vocabulary. On the reading comprehension subtest she was readily able to answer factual questions but experienced difficulty on questions requiring cause–effect reasoning or inferential thinking. Kimberly has a history of difficulty in the area of arithmetic. Her mathematics skills were shown to be compromised in the area of mathematics calculation and, to a lesser extent, in mathematics reasoning. Kimberly showed particular difficulty in her ability to perform mathematical calculations, with errors generally in higher-level subtraction, multiplication, and division processes and in decimals and fractions. Her errors on the basic calculation problems stemmed generally from misalignment of columns, which is a spatial task, rather than poor knowledge of math facts. On the spelling test she showed age-appropriate skills, with errors that were phonetically correct. Her handwriting was neat and legible on the written expression subtest. Her essay showed difficulty with organization and planning and elaboration of ideas. However, her punctuation, capitalization, and grammar were good.

Motor Functioning

Kimberly's performance on the Grooved Pegboard test, a measure of fine motor speed and coordination, was significantly below average in motor functioning with the right and left hands. This test provides measures of motor quickness as well as errors. Scores are converted to z scores, with average performance between -1.0 and $+1.0$. High positive scores are desirable. Kimberly used her left hand as her preferred hand on this task. Her scores were as follows:

Hand	Time	z score
Dominant (left)	100 seconds	-4.72
Nondominant	140 seconds	-9.02
	Dropped pegs	z score
Dominant	2	-6.52
Nondominant	3	-10.34

The Finger Tapping test requires the child to use the index finger on a tapper and tap as quickly as possible for 10 seconds. Average scores reflect adequate finger dexterity. Kimberly used her left hand as her preferred hand on this task. Her scores were as follows:

Dominant hand	35	Average for her age
Nondominant hand	35	Average for her age

Although Kimberly scored in the average range for her age on this task, she experienced significant motor overflow on the task. It was very difficult for her to contain movement in her other fingers (which were to remain still and on the board), and the movement spread to her arm and shoulder as the task progressed. It appears that Kimberly has motor difficulties on these tasks, particularly with her left hand, which is controlled by the right side of her brain. Motor overflow as seen on the Finger Tapping test may imply a compromised CNS, particularly on the right side.

Visual–Perceptual Functioning

The Bender–Gestalt test was administered. This is a measure of the child's ability to copy increasingly more complex figures. Kimberly made 0 errors on this measure. Her figures were well drawn and organized by number on the page.

The JLO requires the child to match 2 lines to an array of 11 lines and measures visual–spatial skills. Kimberly obtained a score of 16 correct, which is significantly below average (average = 26.1 ± 3.5) and consistent with her performance on the DAS.

Executive Functioning

The WCST is a measure of executive or frontal lobe functioning, including the ability to form concepts, generate an organizational strategy, and use examiner feedback to shift strategy to the changing demands of the task. Kimberly's performance is summarized below.

No. of Categories Completed	6	Average to above average
% Perseverative Errors	4%	Above average
Failure to Maintain Set	0	Average to above average

Kimberly performed at the average to above average level on this task, indicating strengths in her cognitive flexibility, problem-solving ability, and response to feedback.

The Conceptual Formation and Analysis and Synthesis subtests of the WJ-R were administered to further evaluate Kimberly's problem-solving skills. She performed fairly well on the initial portion of the task but experienced difficulty as it became more complex and required additional skills in memory. Average scores range from 85 to 115. Kimberly's scores were as follows:

Concept Formation	85
Analysis and Synthesis	79

Behavioral and Emotional Functioning

Kimberly's adjustment was assessed through responses to the BASC, which yields information about perceived cognitive, emotional, familial, and interpersonal problems, as well as parental test-taking attitudes. Kimberly's mother served as informant. *T* scores are reported in the following table, with an average of 50 and an average range of 40 to 60. Lower scores are desirable for the clinical scales, and higher scores are desirable for the adaptive scales. Kimberly's scores were as follows:

	T score	Percentile
Hyperactivity	46	37
Aggression	55	74
Conduct Problems	43	28
Externalizing Problems	48	47
Anxiety	50	59
Depression	42	22
Somatization	64[a]	92
Internalizing Problems	52	67
Atypicality	59	84
Withdrawal	41	16
Attention Problems	68[a]	95
Behavioral Symptoms Index	55	72
Social Skills	52	56
Leadership	48	41
Adaptive Skills Composite	50	49

[a]At-risk behaviors.

According to the parental form of the BASC, Kimberly does not show significant externalizing, internalizing, or adaptive behavioral difficulties. Mild elevations are present on the scales measuring attention and somatization. The somatization scale is artificially elevated because of Kimberly's physical difficulties. Attentional problems appear to be a concern, as reported during the clinical interview. Both Kimberly and her mother indicate that she experiences difficulty with focusing and sustaining her attention, with organization, with overcoming distractibility, and with following through on instructions. Both reported that these difficulties were present prior to the accident; her mother also expressed concern with Kimberly's lethargy and lack of energy, which appeared following the accident.

Kimberly's teacher also completed the BASC, and the following scores were obtained:

Domain	T score	Percentile
Hyperactivity	40	10
Aggression	41	12
Conduct Problems	49	67
Externalizing Problems	43	24
Anxiety	40	15
Depression	44	37
Somatization	45	43
Internalizing Problems	42	21
Attention Problems	68[b]	95
Learning Problems	53	67
School Problems	54	68
Atypicality	45	41
Withdrawal	75[a]	97
Behavioral Symptoms Index	42	25

For the following scales, higher scores are desirable:

Social Skills	33[b]	4
Leadership	36[b]	7
Study Skills	39[b]	16
Adaptive Skills	35[b]	6

[a]Clinical significance; [b]at-risk behaviors.

Difficulty was reported in the areas of social skills, study skills, and attention. Significant concerns were Kimberly's tendency to withdraw from situations that were challenging to her.

The Children's Depression Inventory (CDI) was administered to Kimberly. The CDI requires the child to select statements that are most descriptive of his/her feelings. Kimberly scored in the average range on this measure. She endorsed only two items: "I have to push myself many times to do my schoolwork" and "I have fun at school only once in a while."

The RCMAS is a true–false test; the child reads various statements and determines whether they are true or false of him/her. Kimberly scored well within the average range on all scales. She indicated that she had difficulty with attention on the test.

Kimberly also completed the BASC—Self-Report. T scores are reported in the following table, with an average of 50 and the average range between 40 and 60. Items scoring between 60 and 70 on the BASC are considered "at risk" for the development of further problems. Percentile ranks are also reported.

Domain	T score	Percentile
Attitude to School	68[a]	94
Attitude to Teachers	66[a]	91
School Maladjustment	69[a]	95
Atypicality	57	75
Depression	80[b]	99
Anxiety	57	72
Sense of Inadequacy	67[a]	93
Social Stress	67[a]	93
Clinical Maladjustment	63[a]	89
Emotional Symptoms Index	74[b]	97
For the following scales, higher scores are desirable:		
Relations with Parents	16[b]	2
Interpersonal Relations	18[b]	1
Self-Esteem	40[a]	17
Self-Reliance	36	10
Personal Adjustment	21[b]	2

[a]At-risk behaviors; [b]problem behaviors.

Kimberly's response style on the BASC indicates that she is currently experiencing significant emotional distress both at school and in her overall adjustment. Her ratings indicate that she is feeling most stress in school and that her attitude toward school and teachers is problematic. She does not consider teachers as people who can help her, but that they are unfair and "only look at the bad things you do." Nor does she feel that school is a helpful place, but indicates that she really does not care about school and wants to get out as soon as possible. Kimberly scored in the clinically significant range on the depression subscale, indicating that she frequently feels bad, that no one understands her, that she is always in trouble, and that things are progressively getting worse for her. Adaptively, Kimberly feels that she does not have many friends and that many of her peers tease her and do not like to be around her. She has also expressed concern that she is not living up to her parents' expectations and that they do not think she is doing very well. She feels close to her parents and seeks their approval on her work.

A clinical interview with Kimberly's mother, her teacher, and Kimberly indicated that she does meet DSM-IV criteria for a diagnosis of attention-deficit/hyperactivity disorder: predominantly inattentive type. All reported that Kimberly has difficulty in finishing schoolwork, has problems in paying attention to details, does not seem to listen to what is being said to her, has difficulty in organizing tasks and activities, is forgetful and easily distracted, and often loses her materials. Kimberly endorsed nine symptoms of the possible nine inattention symptoms and only three of the nine hyperactivity/impulsivity symptoms. In addition, her mother reported more lethargy than previously seen, which possibly indicates less arousal.

The Rorschach Inkblot Test was also administered to attempt to uncover areas of emotional functioning that Kimberly would not or could not discuss. Kimberly's protocol indicates that as compared with most children her age she is very responsive to her environment. She has difficulty in separating her feelings from the environmental cues that are present. Like her response on the BASC, Kimberly's protocol indicates that she is experiencing significant distress, which is relatively long-standing and upsetting to her. She does not appear to have the resources to respond to this distress and is presently overwhelmed by her feelings. Such difficulties likely contribute to an inability to change her behavior to match the situation. Kimberly shows relatively little insight into her actions. Moreover, she is unduly optimistic about her ability to cope with problems and appears to ruminate on her shortcomings. However, when overwhelmed by a situation, Kimberly is likely to withdraw from it and may distance herself from others as a protection. Thus, although Kimberly may wish to have support from parents, teachers, and peers, she may resist such support because she does not believe that she can live up to the other person's expectations or because she does not trust that this support will be maintained. Kimberly's Rorschach protocol indicates the presence of a coping deficit as well as depression.

Kimberly was somewhat unwilling to complete the TAT. The TAT requires the child to tell a story about a picture. Her main themes included the hero's being challenged to complete a task. Some of her stories reflected success and happiness, but most involved escaping from a situation or avoiding consequences for misbehavior. There were also themes of disappointment and shame.

Impressions and Recommendations

Kimberly is a 13-year 1-month-old left-handed female who experienced head trauma at age 11 in a motor vehicle accident. She was taken to the emergency room, and a right frontoparietal scalp hematoma was diagnosed with underlying depressed skull fracture, broken ribs, and a lacerated liver. Kimberly was in a coma for 2 weeks and was hospitalized for approximately the next 2½ months receiving occupational, physical, and speech/language therapy. Neuropsychological assessment following the hospitalization found average verbal ability with below-average nonverbal skills. It was reported that the nonverbal learning disability was present before the accident but likely exacerbated by the accident. Memory for visual information appeared to be compromised, and Kimberly was described as disinhibited and impulsive. Gross and fine motor testing by the occupational therapist and physical therapist found significant delays, particularly on Kimberly's left side; balance and gait were determined to be areas of concern. Reevaluation showed good progress, and Kimberly was attending public school with special education services provided. There was continuing concern, however, about Kimberly's attention and motor difficulties. The pediatric neurologist reported that her motor difficulties were most likely "permanent."

School records indicate the presence of concerns about attention, organization, and learning problems, particularly in mathematics, prior to the accident. The findings of a school assessment team 6 months prior to the accident were a learning disability, a need for occupational therapy due to delays in balance, agility, and fine motor skills. Reassessment of Kimberly's cognitive abilities approximately 1 year following the accident found superior verbal ability and a decline in nonverbal ability. Reports of weakness in organizational ability, study skills, and mathematics continued. Some symptoms of anxiety and depression were also reported.

Kimberly's current neuropsychological functioning is generally within age expectations except for motor, memory, and visual–spatial skills. She shows very superior verbal ability with average nonverbal skills. When tests are not timed so as to not penalize Kimberly for lack of motor speed, she performs at a level commensurate with her ability prior to the accident. Significant weakness is present in visual–spatial ability. Achievement testing shows superior reading skills with average spelling ability. Although Kimberly's reading comprehension skills are within average limits, qualitative analysis of her errors indicated difficulty with cause–effect reasoning and inferential thinking. Mathematics skills are significantly below average for Kimberly's ability, and she had particular difficulty in aligning numbers on arithmetic problems—a visual–spatial skill. Kimberly's memory skills are variable, depending on what type of task is presented. When material is presented that is verbal or that involves a pattern that can be verbally mediated, Kimberly performs at age level. Visual memory and facial memory skills are significantly below expectations for her age and ability. Her learning of new material is also influenced by the modality of presentation; that is, Kimberly learns verbal material at a level commensurate with her age mates but does not learn visual material at the same rate as her peers. These findings are consistent with a diagnosis of a nonverbal learning disability. Fine motor skills are significantly below expectations for her age, with more decrement found with the left hand than the right. These findings are consistent with the localization of brain damage resulting from the injury.

Attentional testing indicated mild difficulties with sustained visual attention, particularly when the stimulus was presented less frequently. A behavioral rating scale indicated mild to moderate concern by her mother about Kimberly's attentional abilities.

Emotional assessment indicated the presence of depressive symptoms and Kimberly's sense of being overwhelmed by her feelings. Projective testing indicated that Kimberly is feeling very stressed by the demands of home and school. She also shows a tendency to ruminate over her problems and may worry about her ability to live up to her own and others' expectations. Kimberly indicated concern about her brain being bad and was worried that it might never work as well as it did prior to the accident. These feelings of sadness can certainly exacerbate her attentional difficulties and may interfere with her performance in school.

In summary, Kimberly's learning difficulties, attention problems, and organizational difficulties predate the accident as reported by school records. She shows signs of a nonverbal learning disability (mathematics difficulty, visual–spatial problems), which is also characteristic of her performance prior to the accident. When motor skills are not required for solving a nonverbal task, Kimberly shows age appropriate skills. However, her visual–spatial ability is compromised. Such difficulties are related to a nonverbal learning disability. Both Kimberly's motor skills and visual–spatial skills were problematic prior to the accident and, given the localization of the head injury, are likely to have been exacerbated following the accident. Kimberly has made remarkable progress and no decrement is found in her verbal or nonverbal abilities when tasks are adapted to her physical difficulty.

Because of Kimberly's attention and organizational problems that continue to present challenges to her learning, coupled with her lower arousal as reported by her mother, consideration should be given to medication intervention.

Kimberly also showed signs of dysthymia. Although attentional and depressive symptoms can co-occur, it is important for both issues to be addressed in treatment. It appears appropriate for Kimberly to enter into individual psychotherapy to assist with her ability to cope with her difficulties and to discuss her fears about her future capabilities.

CHAPTER 7

◆◆◆

Promoting Reentry into the School Setting

◆

Assessment is an important part of a child's successful reentry into school. It is only the first step, however. As discussed in Chapter 5, the IDEA and Section 504 provide for services for children with TBI. A recent study found that school professionals have difficulty in determining which children with TBI are eligible for services (Clark, 1996). To complicate matters further, individual states are inconsistent as to how eligibility for services can be determined. Although the definition of TBI as stated in Public Law 101-476 excludes children experiencing difficulty due to internal causes, some states include these children (Katsiyannis & Conderman, 1994). In addition, children who have experienced brain damage due to drowning are included, whereas those who have experienced brain trauma due to electrocution, cardiac arrest, or anesthetic accidents are not (Clark, 1996).

It is estimated that 20% of children with head injuries will require some special education services because of residual disability (Kraus et al., 1990). These children generally have experienced moderate to severe head injuries. According to the literature, it is not uncommon for a child to have been receiving special education services prior to the injury (Levin et al., 1994). In this case it is very important to reassess the child's needs based on new information and to adjust the IEP accordingly.

A range of placements can be available for a child with TBI. Some children cannot be discharged directly from the hospital and may require residential placement. Others may need homebound instruction because of the severity of their injuries. For still other children, special education classes may be required. Such classes vary from self-contained settings to inclusion. In many cases a child will require a stepwise transition to the school, possibly beginning with a half-day placement and increasing the length of the

111

school day as the child shows readiness. A study by Rosen and Gerring (1986) found that 10% of children with TBI required home instruction, 11% a reduced or modified school program, 20% special education programs, 10% residential placement, and 14% were unable to return to school because of an ongoing comatose state. This study also found that 18% did not require any special education services.

The timing of return to school is an important variable for successful reentry. It is recommended that prior to returning to school, the child be able to function within a school setting and able to respond to instruction (Clark, 1996). The ability to attend to simultaneous input from several modalities (i.e., tactile, vision, hearing) and to work unassisted for 30 minutes or longer has been found to be indicative of readiness for school reentry (Mira & Tyler, 1991). Key skills that appear to be required for reentry to a classroom include (1) ability to attend to classroom instruction, (2) ability to understand and retain information, (3) ability to reason and express ideas, (4) ability to solve problems, (5) ability to plan and monitor one's own performance, and (6) self-control (Cohen, 1996).

Successful reentry requires a great deal of planning, which should begin once the school receives notice that a child has sustained a brain injury. A smooth transition from hospital/rehabilitation center to school requires that all participants be informed of the skills in which the child/adolescent is currently proficient as well as those that may develop at a later time.

Interagency cooperation has been found to be imperative for the successful reentry of the child into the school system (Carney & Gerring, 1990). Communication between agencies, however, can be hindered by a lack of common vocabulary between professionals (Farmer et al., 1996). It has been suggested that this communication begin when the child is first hospitalized and continue throughout recovery (DePompei & Blosser, 1993; Janus, 1994). It is important for the school personnel to be conversant with medical terminology. Such ongoing information sharing provides a platform for the development of appropriate goals and objectives for the IEP. The IEP, developed over the course of hospitalization and discharge, must include the current levels of performance, goals and objectives (short- and long-term), need for related services (OT, PT, speech and language), the anticipated duration of services, and methods for evaluation of the child's progress (Carter & Savage, 1985).

A formal planning meeting is generally held at the end of the child's hospitalization or rehabilitation stay. It is important for school professionals to be present at this meeting, but they should not expect an automatic invitation. Continuing contact with parents and medical personnel is important to ensure a smooth transition. Medical personnel often rely on parents to let the school know that a meeting is being scheduled. When communication has been ongoing during a child's hospitalization, it is less likely that the school will be left out of the planning.

As information is gathered, it may be helpful for the team of professionals to have a summary sheet providing the most important information as to the child's functioning. Most of the information requested in Table 7.1 is included in the child's medical file, and most parents are more than willing to release such records to school professionals. However, medical records are notoriously difficult to read, and it is time-consuming to attempt to find the relevant material when writing a report. Table 7.1 is an

TABLE 7.1. Intake Sheet for School Reentry

Child's name: DOB: Age:

Parent: Phone:

Date of TBI: Hospital:

Hospital contact and phone number:

Level of TBI: Mild   Moderate   Severe

Length of coma: Length of PTA:

Location of brain injury:

Date of hospital discharge:

Date(s) of neuropsychological evaluation(s):

Results of other evaluations conducted:

Prior special education services? If yes, what category and level of service?

Prior academic and cognitive strengths and weaknesses?

Prior behavioral and social functioning levels?

Current health issues
   Seizure disorder?
   Medications?
   Visual and hearing skills
   Balance/mobility
   Fine motor/gross motor
Current level of functioning
   Language
   Memory
   Cognitive
   Achievement
   Behavior
   Social skills/peer relationships
Current related services and amount of time
   Occupational therapy
   Physical therapy
   Speech and language therapy
   Psychological counseling
   Family counseling

example of a summary sheet that may be helpful to school personnel in compiling data and completing a multidisciplinary report. This information may be completed when key school personnel attend the discharge meeting at the hospital or rehabilitation clinic. It is also an example of why it is imperative to maintain communication with the family so that the scheduling of these meetings is available to school personnel.

The meeting held prior to termination of medical services provides an opportunity to gather information as to the child's level of functioning as well as recommendations for his/her continued care. In addition, this meeting may be the one time that all concerned professionals are in attendance, and it is important for school personnel to ask questions in order to assist with transition. They can ask about recommendations for a half or full day of school, medications and their side effects, therapy required, emotional and behavioral functioning, physical accommodations that may be needed, and methods that have been successful in working with the child. A plan for additional communication among team members should also be developed at this meeting. Ongoing communication is particularly important if a child's progress is not proceeding as anticipated (Farmer et al., 1996).

It can be intimidating to sit in one of these meetings with professionals who are used to working with each other and who seem to speak another language. However, it is imperative that you speak up and ask questions in regard to the reintegration of the child into the usual school setting. It is also important to determine the additional services that will be provided to the child through the early stages of his/her school reentry.

Families may experience difficulty with the transition to school, as well as with a child's ongoing hospitalization. Research has indicated that families who were dysfunctional prior to the accident remain so after the accident; in some instances the dysfunction actually increases. Moreover, families who were relatively underinvolved prior to the accident may experience additional difficulty in accessing or wanting community supports (Waaland et al., 1993). For the transition to be successful, it has been strongly recommended that an interagency individualized family plan be developed (DePompei & Blosser, 1993). Such a plan would include documentation of the family's needs and resources as well as the supports that can be provided. These efforts have been found to pay off in the long run, in terms of sustained communication between agencies to promote the child's recovery to the fullest potential (Blosser & DePompei, 1994; Farmer et al., 1996).

The school professionals who should be involved in such planning meetings include the school psychologist, related services therapists as needed (OT, PT, speech and language), the school nurse, and special education and regular education teachers. It is important that a school case manager be appointed so that services can be coordinated efficiently. Family members should also be in attendance, and, as appropriate, the child or adolescent may benefit from attending as well. The level of comfort of the child or adolescent in attending the meeting must be considered in deciding on such attendance.

The IEP may be written during the planning meeting or at a separate meeting at the school. To develop the most appropriate IEP, certain questions must be answered by the medical staff and/or rehabilitation teachers. Questions that are particularly important for the development of the IEP and successful school reentry are listed in Table 7.2. It will not be possible to answer some of the questions until the child has returned to school, and others may require an interview with the homebound teacher or the teachers in the rehabilitation unit.

Once the planning meeting has been conducted for a child reentering school, it is important to begin preparing for reentry at the child's school. The child's needs throughout the day must be considered. Because of the common finding that children with TBI are most productive early in the day, challenging classes should be scheduled early.

As discussed in Chapter 5, achievement tests may show few difficulties in the child's learning as compared with the problems seen in the classroom. To properly plan for the child's reentry into school, it is imperative to evaluate not only performance on standardized tests but also information gathered during hospitalization as to the child's learning style and learning needs (Savage, 1991). In addition, although children with TBI have been found to score within an age-appropriate range on these tests, the problem-solving skills they use to obtain such scores differ significantly from those of peers (Fay et al., 1994). For example, one child was able to show age-appropriate reading comprehension skills on the WIAT during a screening upon return to school. Her performance in the classroom was significantly below this level, and the teacher and school psychologist were puzzled by the discrepancy. Upon questioning the child as to how she arrived at the correct answers, it was discovered that she was using her fund of information to answer the questions—not the passage she was to have read.

Related services also need to be scheduled during a time the child is most productive (Clark, 1996). Early release from classes may be necessary, particularly for children with motor and sensory deficits. As appropriate, school staff should be informed about the child's needs, including the school secretary, custodian, lunch personnel, and bus driver.

SYSTEMS ISSUES IN SCHOOL REENTRY

Systems issues are beginning to be understood as constituting one of the main predictors for good outcomes for children with TBI and other dis-

TABLE 7.2. Questions for Reentry to School

Area of concern	Suggested questions to be asked
Cognitive/ intellectual	1. How does the child learn new material? 2. Are attentional problems present that interfere? 3. Are comprehension difficulties present? 4. Does the child process information more slowly than most of his/ her age mates? 5. Is the child's learning affected by time of day? 6. Are there problems with short- and long-term memory? 7. Does the child profit from repetition or from teaching of memory strategies? 8. Does the child recall meaningful or nonmeaningful material more readily? 9. Does the child appear to learn better visually or orally? 10. Is there difficulty with organization and planning skills? 11. Can the child break tasks down into smaller parts?
Language skills	1. Does the child experience difficulty expressing him/herself? 2. Is there a problem with understanding what he/she has heard? 3. Are articulation problems present? 4. How many directions can the child follow at one time? 5. What happens when the child is unable to communicate? Are there behavioral difficulties, withdrawal, etc.?
Achievement	1. Is the child able to take notes during a lecture? 2. Are assistive technology devices needed? 3. Can the child process information at the same rate as his/her peers? 4. Do timed tests prevent the child from achieving up to his/her potential? 5. Does the child become distracted when too much stimulation is present? 6. Do tests have to be administered individually, orally, or through another modality? 7. What is the recommended length of day? 8. What are the instructional priorities for this child? 9. Is special education appropriate for this child? 10. Which classes are anticipated to be more difficult for this child? Which ones easier? 11. What is the best balance of classes—reading vs. hands-on? 12. Does the child require special education or Section 504?
Motor and physical	1. What adaptations are necessary to the physical plant? Are the bathrooms accessible? 2. What types of physical education classes are appropriate for this child? 3. What amount of time can this child profit from in school—half day, full day? 4. Is special transportation to and from school required? 5. Is help required during lunch hour? 6. Does the child's desk have to be adjusted in any manner? 7. Is special seating required?

TABLE 7.2.	*(continued)*

Behavior	1. Does the child's behavior require any special considerations?
	2. What classroom modifications are required for success? More or less structure?
	3. How is the child coping with his/her deficits?
	4. Has the child had any contact with peers through hospitalization?
	5. What are the expectations for the child's peer relationships?
	6. Does the child need a counselor or psychologist to assist with the transition and to help with organizational questions and coping?
	7. What medications are being used, and what are their side effects/benefits?
Relationships between parent and school	1. What is the family's understanding of the brain–behavior relationships now seen in their child?
	2. How is the family coping with the deficits now seen?
	3. How has communication from your child's doctors been provided during the hospitalization and rehabilitation? What has been successful in this process, and what should be avoided?
	4. Do the parents have an understanding of the school's responsibility, and are they aware of their right to educational services?
	5. Have the parents been provided with information as to community resources to assist in the transition?

abling conditions (McKee & Witt, 1990; Ylvisaker et al., 1993). Among these issues are teacher qualities, peer interactions, and the environment of the school (Farmer & Peterson, 1995). It is increasingly clear that teachers require additional training in order for the reentering child to be fully integrated (Midgley et al., 1989). A child's returning to school can be quite intimidating, both for the child and for the teacher. A teacher may not feel prepared to work with a child with TBI and may be fearful of seizures or of harming the child even in the usual classroom routine.

Inservice for key personnel appears to be essential and should be a responsibility of the IEP team (Mira & Tyler, 1991). A workshop should be held to provide information about brain injury and the individual child's strengths and weaknesses. Any required modifications should be explained in detail, and an opportunity for discussion of additional concerns should be provided to dispel any myths or misunderstandings about TBI.

Teachers

One of the key predictors for successful reentry is the teacher's acceptance of the child's reentry and placement in his/her classroom (Rosen & Gerring, 1986). Children with TBI show as much variability in behavior and ability as typically developing children. Children with TBI who are likable and whose families are easy to get along with are most readily accepted; others may not be so fortunate. For example, a child who is oppositional and defiant may actually push help away and school personnel may be less willing to provide additional assistance. Likewise, challenging and aggressive parents may also be avoided rather than provided support. For these children it is important to use the adaptations begun in the hospital. Appropriate management in the hospital has been found to be predictive of later adjustment in school when these procedures are shared (Papas, 1993). In addition, the support of the administration and the case manager is particularly important for the teacher to feel empowered to work with the child. Additional time for planning, paraprofessional support, and the support of the multidisciplinary team are all important to assist the teacher and to ensure the child's adjustment. Support from school-based instructional teams has been found to increase communication among a school's staff and to improve the delivery of services (Mercer & Mercer, 1989; Smith, 1991).

A teacher must also be informed that he/she is one of the most important people in the child's recovery. Any child, even one who attends for only a short period of the day, may feel empowered by his/her reentry and become more hopeful about his/her eventual recovery (Cohen, 1996). The teacher can assist the child in evaluating his/her improvement over time and provide encouragement to try tasks that are challenging but doable. In this manner, a child's self-esteem can be boosted through successful reentry.

It is important for school staff to recognize that the program for a child with TBI frequently changes, depending on the child's progress and evolving needs. Thus, sharing information across the school's resource team is crucial. Particularly important is the juxtaposition of special education resources and mainstreaming. For some children with TBI a more structured learning environment may be required for continued progress—ongoing evaluation can answer this question (National Joint Committee on Learning Disabilities, 1992; Silver, 1991).

There are also some key behaviors that can be readily misinterpreted by school personnel not familiar with TBI. Such interpretation can lead to inappropriate placement decisions. A child who has problems with expressive language may have difficulty explaining concepts that he/she truly understands. Such difficulty may be misinterpreted to indicate that the child is a "slow learner." It is important that the teacher provide opportunities for the child to demonstrate his/her learning by other means, rather than solely using words. In addition, a child's problems in processing information may reflect difficulty in cognitive development, rather than a lower IQ. A teacher looking for strengths and weaknesses in the processing of information may assist the child in developing skills to compensate for these difficulties. As the child progresses, his/her ability to manage behavior and develop skills increases. Although children with TBI often show amazing gains in the first year following recovery, slower recovery can occur up to 5 years after injury (Teeter & Semrud-Clikeman, 1997).

Learning Environments

Learning environments should be repeatedly assessed in regard to the child's ability to function appropriately. Various environments can interact with task demands to assist the child or to make progress very difficult. A child's skills will fluctuate over time, and when a child repeatedly fails in one or more areas, the educational program should be reevaluated. Table 7.3 illustrates various environments and task demands.

In some instances, additional individual support may be necessary for the child to profit from instruction, whereas in others classroom assistance can be provided. Emerging evidence indicates that for some children, integration of the various prescribed therapies into actual school activities is most successful for later learning. Using actual classroom materials during therapy may be the most appropriate and fruitful approach (Smith, 1991). One of the concerns with pull-out programs (which require the child to leave the classroom for therapy) is the decrease in time in the regular classroom. For students requiring several therapies, time in the classroom can be

TABLE 7.3. Learning Environments and Task Demands

Learning environment	Task demands
Structured or unstructured	• Is there a difference in behavior and task completion? • Does the child perform better when materials are given as a whole or in pieces?
Independent versus teacher-led work	• Does the child experience difficulty completing work that is not teacher-led? • Is the difficulty due to attention, speed, or handwriting deficits? • Is there an optimal amount of time that the child can direct his/her own work? • Is there any difference between subjects as to work completion? Math versus reading?
Ability to profit from classroom instruction	• Does the child perform better when material is visual in nature? • Does a problem with memory appear to interfere with learning? • Does the child retain the information from day to day?

substantially decreased, making progress difficult. For this reason, therapists should consult with the child's teacher to determine the optimal amount of time for therapy and may consider providing some therapies within the classroom itself.

INDIVIDUALIZED TRANSITION PLAN

Bergland (1996) recommends a developmental approach in implementing a program. For younger children, time is available for compensation and learning. For older adolescents, injury may interfere with normal developmental transitions, necessitating additional support for adjustment. Thus, for the adolescent the transition to the adult world may be more problematic, and a transition plan, as required by Public Law 101-476 (IDEA), will have to be developed. Like an IEP, an appropriate Individualized Transition Plan (ITP) includes a relevant assessment of the adolescent's needs, as well as consideration of the type of instruction required, needs for daily living, community resources, employment, and a vocational evaluation (Baxter et al., 1985; Cook et al., 1987). Linkages to community services must be explored when the child approaches the age of 14 and continued through age 16, depending on the individual adolescent's needs. The timing of this plan is dependent on the severity of the adolescent's needs and his/her prognosis for future vocational functioning. These linkages become particularly important as the child prepares to leave the school environment, generally between the ages of 18 and 21. Wehman (1992) suggests that there must be linkages at the local and state levels; Minnesota and Kansas provide models for such linkages. For example, in St. Paul, Minnesota, the Project Explore program is a curriculum-based transition plan designed to be used at training sites for adolescents with head injury (Gaylord, 1991). This project explores the adolescent's functioning, using an assessment of work-related behavior, work and academic skills, and behavior over a 6-month period. This assessment then serves as a baseline for improvement and continued support in specific areas. It also provides a plan for functioning after high school.

Linkages to state vocational workers are particularly relevant for adolescents with TBI because the case manager for the school system is generally no longer available. For adolescents entering the workforce, adjustments to the workplace may be required and a state case worker from a state's Department of Vocational Rehabilitation can be very helpful. Some adolescents are able and motivated to attend college, and they should be linked up with the Office for Students with Disabilities at the university or college chosen for attendance. Such a transition should be started prior to entry into college so that interventions are available immediately. Bergland

(1996) suggests the following areas be explored for entry to postsecondary education.

Physical accessibility
Faculty/staff awareness
Existence of academic supports (peer note takers, computers, etc.)
Availability of syllabi and lecture notes
Flexibility in test administration
Opportunity for social interactions
Availability of counseling
Availability of career and vocational counseling

It is also suggested that the transition be smoothed through interaction between the school system and the college/university disability team. Particular importance is placed on the ability of the adolescent to enter the social networks for a good college experience, an area found to be particularly problematic for many adolescents with TBI (Holmes, 1988). A student's taking classes before the end of high school at the college/university (if local) may assist in the transition to a new setting. Enrollment in classes that stress study strategies may also be very helpful to adolescents with TBI; this approach has been found to be successful in Missouri and Texas (Holmes, 1988).

For adolescents entering the workforce from high school, the transition can be difficult, and the involvement of various agencies is particularly important (Bergland, 1996). Continuing in high school until age 21 may be the best option for adolescents with severe and ongoing impairment. Hands-on work experience can be invaluable in providing a smoother transition and an appropriate evaluation of the adolescent's work skills. The use of task analysis to determine the adolescent's ability to function independently has been found to be quite helpful in this process (Calub et al., 1989). Such an assessment involves the adolescent's ability to process information quickly, to handle frustration and ambiguous situations, and to manage social situations, as well as the usual evaluation of cognitive and learning skills. It has been recommended that a job coach be available in the work setting to provide support for skill development over time (West et al., 1991). It has also been found that adolescents with TBI may "fail" in the first job placement, but if planning and involvement of the job coach are continued to the second placement, success is more likely (Bergland, 1996). The use of such a work-study experience in high school has been related to later mastery and to successful reintegration into the workforce.

Thus, involvement of the school in providing support for children and adolescents requires a great deal of planning to be successful. In addition, it is important for school personnel, particularly the school psychologist and/

or school counselor, to be aware of state and local supports for children with vocational needs beyond the school setting. Developmental issues become quite important for both the younger child and, particularly, for the adolescent in such planning. A case study of a child's reentry into school may illustrate the pitfalls and the concerns that can arise.

CASE STUDY

The following is a neuropsychological report and the recommendations developed by the school following this assessment.

Background Information

Sally was a 6-year 6-month-old female when she was hit by a baseball bat during a family reunion. She was unconscious when the emergency medical team arrived. Medical records indicate that she had a low Glasgow Coma Scale (GCS) rating of 4 upon admission to an area hospital. She was subsequently intubated. Seizure activity was noted, which was treated with Ativan and Cerebryx. A CT scan of her head indicated a right orbital fracture as well as pneumocephalus and subarachnoid blood. Subsequently, swelling of the left frontal scalp and a right perifocal hematoma were found. CT was repeated and showed a right frontal contusion and fractures to her cranial vault. During the next 2 weeks Sally improved and began speaking. She had difficulty with memory for short-term information, as noted by the ward nurses in the medical records. Balance difficulties were also noticed, which continued upon discharge 3 days later. She began complaining of headaches, averaging about three a week and generally occurring after she had played hard. Balance continued to be an area of concern, as well as a tendency to talk about an unrelated subject during a conversation. This behavior had not been present prior to the accident.

Sally was provided homebound instruction for the remainder of the school year—approximately 6 weeks. Her tutor reported that Sally had "caught up" and had passed the mastery tests. Repetition of first grade was not recommended nor was summer school. She was to begin second grade in the fall without any special education services. Sally had not been evaluated prior to the accident nor during her recovery. No medication had been prescribed.

Developmental History

Sally lives with her biological parents, younger sister, and older brother. She was the result of a normal pregnancy and delivery. She met her developmental milestones within normal limits, and her mother describes her development as normal. Until the accident Sally was reported to be relatively healthy. She wears glasses for nearsightedness. Sally was also reported to make friends easily and to have a generally good temperament. Her mother says that Sally's attention span has declined since her accident. No problems have been noted in school, and her teachers report that she is doing as expected for a first grader.

Current Concerns

An evaluation was requested by Sally's mother. She was concerned because Sally was showing difficulties with memory and attention—difficulties that had not been present prior to the accident. No psychological or neuropsychological evaluation had been completed, and she wished for a measure of Sally's performance. She was also concerned because the school did not think there were any difficulties in learning. However, Sally was having to spend 3 to 4 hours each night on her homework, and it seemed as if reteaching of basic skills was continually needed.

Behavioral Observations

Sally was accompanied to the testing sessions by her mother and older brother. Because of her fatigue, the assessment was broken into 2 days of 3 hours each. She readily joined the examiner and was cooperative, friendly, and open throughout the sessions. Her affect was full and her mood was good. Her language was well developed, and she was readily able to express her thoughts. She showed good attention through most of the testing.

Sally frequently misheard words that are similar in sound (*drapes/grapes*, *web/wed*). She was quite distracted by articles in the room but easily redirected to the task at hand. Sally's right hand was observed to have a tremor that at times made it difficult for her to write. She told the examiner that her hand sometimes makes her mad because it "doesn't work good." The following results are believed to be a valid and reliable representation of her current level of functioning.

Test Results and Interpretation

Tests Administered

The following tests were administered: The Wechsler Intelligence Scale for Children—Third Edition (WISC-III), Stanford–Binet Intelligence Scale—IV (memory and copying subtests), Wechsler Individual Achievement Test (WIAT), Woodcock Reading Mastery Test—Revised, California Verbal

Learning Test—Children's Version (CVLT-C), Wisconsin Card Sorting Test (WCST), Beery Developmental Test of Visual–Motor Integration (VMI), Purdue Pegboard, Finger Tapping, and Behavior Assessment System for Children (BASC)—Parent Form, Clinical Interview.

Cognitive Functioning

The WISC-III is a measure of basic cognitive development. The verbal subtests measure the child's ability to understand and use language, and the performance subtests evaluate the child's skills in perceptual organization and understanding visual information. Average standard scores range from 85 to 115, and average scaled scores range from 7 to 13. Sally's scores were as follows:

Verbal IQ	102
Performance IQ	100
Full scale IQ	101

Information	9	Picture Completion	6
Similarities	10	Coding	9
Arithmetic	13	Picture Arrangement	9
Vocabulary	12	Block Design	12
Comprehension	8	Object Assembly	14
Digit Span	9	Symbol Search	7

Sally achieved a full scale IQ of 101, which places her in the average range of intellectual functioning and at the 53rd national percentile. There is a 95% probability that Sally's true score falls between 97 and 107. Both Sally's verbal IQ (VIQ) of 102 (55%) and her performance IQ (PIQ) of 100 (50%) are within this range. On the verbal subtests Sally showed average ability for her age in her fund of general information, abstract reasoning, short-term auditory memory for digits, and one-word vocabulary development. Above average performance was noted on a measure of arithmetic reasoning skills. On the performance subtests Sally showed average skills in visual–motor speed and on a measure of visual reasoning. Superior strength was found in perceptual organization. Weakness was found on a measure of attention to detail and on speed of information processing.

Achievement Functioning

The WIAT is a measure of general academic functioning in the areas of reading, arithmetic, and writing. On the reading subtests the child is asked to read single words and then to read a passage and answer questions about its content. On the arithmetic subtests the child is asked to solve word problems and general calculation problems. The writing subtests require the child to spell words and then to write a story on a topic. Average standard scores are between 85 and 115. Sally's scores were as follows (grade norms are in parentheses):

	Standard score	Percentile
Basic reading	100 (85)	53
Reading Comprehension	100 (84)	50
Reading Composite	100 (84)	50
Mathematics Reasoning	89 (76)	23
Numerical Operations	103 (84)	58
Mathematics Composite	93 (77)	32
Spelling	95 (79)	37

Standard scores for both grade and age were calculated because Sally is one of the younger second graders. Based on age, Sally is achieving within expectations in all academic areas. Slight weakness was noted in her ability to understand quantity (Which number is bigger?) and to identify more difficult shapes (cubes, pyramids). When Sally's skills are calculated for her grade placement, she shows delays in mathematics reasoning and spelling skills. These areas must be addressed by her teacher to make sure that Sally understands the basic concepts behind the operations. An additional test of reading was conducted to evaluate Sally's individual skills. The Woodcock Reading Mastery Test—Revised evaluates the child's ability to read single words, sound out nonsense words, and comprehend a passage. Sally's scores were as follows:

	Standard score	Percentile
Letter Identification	97	41
Word Identification	100	49
Word Attack	90	25
Passage Comprehension	98	44

There were no significant areas of weakness. However, the examiner did note that Sally does much better when a visual cue is provided with an auditory direction.

Memory and Learning

The CVLT-C was administered to assess Sally's ability to learn verbal material after several exposures. The task also provides measures of recall and recognition of previously learned material. Sally's scores on this measure are listed in the following table. Scores have a mean of 0, with standard scores of −1.0 to +1.0 indicating performance within the broad average range.

	Raw score	z score
List A, Trial 1	4	−0.5
List A, Trial 5	4	−1.5
Trials 1 to 5	24	38
List B, Free Recall	5	−0.5
List A, Short Delay Free Recall	5	−0.5
List A, Short Delay Cued Recall	9	1.0
List A, Long Delay Free Recall	2	−2.0
List A, Long Delay Cued Recall	4	−1.0
Correct Recognition Hits	14	0.5
Discriminability	77.78%	−0.5
Learning Slope	0.0	−1.5

Sally's performance on the CVLT-C indicates that she has adequate initial ability to encode information in working memory. She shows difficulty in retaining information even when it is repeated over several trials. She does show ability to utilize memory strategies, however, and her performance improved when such strategies where provided to her. Sally's ability to recall information also improves when she is asked to recognize the information rather than trying to recall it spontaneously.

The findings from the memory measures have important implications for Sally's school performance. First, Sally displays below average ability to learn new information through repeated exposure without the aid of concrete cues. Therefore, in the classroom she will most likely learn material at a much slower rate than other children. She does not spontaneously generate efficient strategies for encoding and may have to be taught more effective means of remembering new material. It also appears that new learning may be taking place but that Sally is having difficulty with retrieval. Thus, she should be provided with a system of cueing herself to help her to remember information she has just learned. Moreover, new learning should be rehearsed often to make retrieval somewhat easier.

Additional memory testing was conducted using the Stanford–Binet Intelligence Scale—IV. Average subtest scores on this test range from 42 to 58 and average composite scores from 84 to 116.

Bead Memory	35
Memory for Sentences	46
Memory for Digits	44
Memory for Objects	45
Short-Term Memory	81

Sally shows age-appropriate skills in recalling information that is visual or provided through context (memory for sentences). She experienced difficulty on Bead Memory, a subtest that required her to sequence beads. Sally recalled the correct beads but generally confused the sequence she needed to replicate.

Executive Functioning

The WCST is a measure of executive functioning, including the ability to form concepts, generate an organizational strategy, and use examiner feedback to shift strategy according to the changing demands of the task. Sally's performance is summarized here:

Categories Achieved	5	Normal range = 3
Failure to Maintain Set	2	Normal range = 2–4

Standard Score (100 + 15)	
Total Errors	87
Perseverative Errors	105
Nonperseverative Errors	85

Sally exhibited average ability to generate good strategies on this measure, correctly achieving five of six categories. She was able to flexibly adapt her responses to the demands of the task and to use examiner feedback to learn from her mistakes.

Visual–Motor Functioning

On the Purdue Pegboard test, a measure of fine motor speed and coordination, Sally achieved significantly below-average performance with her right hand and with both hands, but normal performance with her left hand. Average z scores range from +1.00 to –1.00.

Hand	Number of pegs	z score
Dominant (right)	8	–2.46
Nondominant	11	+0.38
Both Hands	4	–2.39

The Finger Tapping test requires the child to tap as quickly as possible for 10 seconds. It is believed to be a measure of fine motor speed and coordination. It is expected that the dominant hand will be faster than the nondominant hand. Sally showed significantly below average performance with her right hand and slightly below average performance with her left hand. It is expected that the nondominant hand would be approximately 10% slower than the dominant one.

Hand	Number of taps	z score
Dominant (right)	26	–1.75
Nondominant	26	–1.19

These findings indicate that Sally's right hand (left side of the motor strip of her brain) is not functioning within expectations for her age. Because there was swelling on the left side of her head, some damage may have occurred that accounts for this difficulty. The tremors noticed were more significant on this task than when Sally's hand was at rest and more remarkable in the right hand than the left.

The VMI measures visual–motor skills by having the child copy increasingly complex geometric shapes and designs. Sally obtained a standard score of 73 on this measure, indicating that her visual–motor integration falls significantly below expectations for her age. Sally had difficulty in copying the more complex figures, particularly in integrating more than one part. The copying subtest of the Stanford–Binet was also administered, and on this task Sally scored within age expectations. The difference between the two tasks was the complexity of the designs. Thus, when complexity increases, Sally experiences ever more difficulty in integrating the material as well as in copying it.

Behavioral Functioning

Sally's mother also completed the BASC, an integrated system designed to facilitate the differential diagnosis and classification of a variety of emotional and behavioral disorders of children and to aid in the design of treatment plans. Her responses on this measure were consistent with her report of Sally's behavior in her interview and with school reports. T scores are reported in the following table, with an average of 50 and the average range between 40 and 60. Scores between 60 and 70 on the BASC are considered "at risk" indicators for the development of further problems. Percentile ranks are also reported.

Domain	T score	Percentile
Hyperactivity	47	43
Aggression	44	27
Conduct Problems	41	15
Externalizing Problems	43	24
Anxiety	42	24
Depression	39	10
Somatization	50	58
Internalizing Problems	42	22
Atypicality	40	16
Withdrawal	44	31
Attention Problems	53	67
Behavioral Symptoms Index	42	21
Adaptability	44	28
Social Skills	53	61
Leadership	51	55
Adaptive Skills Composite	49	46

Sally's mother did not report any clinically significant symptoms and said that her daughter is performing well both in her behavior and in her emotional functioning.

Sally's teacher also completed the BASC form. No areas were identified as clinically significant. A slight elevation (*T* score of 60) was found in attention difficulties, basically in the areas of distractibility and difficulty in completing tasks on time.

Impressions and Recommendations

Sally is a 6-year 11-month-old female who experienced TBI approximately 5 months ago. Injury was sustained in the right frontal area, and her mother reported that another fracture was found in the posterior section of her brain. Sally has a bright and sparkling personality and is cooperative and willing to try difficult tasks. Her recovery from the accident has been very good, according to medical and parental reports. Some difficulty remains in Sally's attention and in her tendency to insert unrelated material into conversations. Her teachers have reported adequate academic progress, and she has just begun the second grade. This evaluation found average ability with strengths in arithmetic reasoning and perceptual organization. Weaknesses were found in Sally's ability to process information quickly and in her attention to detail. Academically, Sally is progressing as expected for her age. However, as compared with her grade placement, there are weaknesses in mathematics understanding and in spelling. Her reading skills are at age level.

In all cases Sally performed better when a visual clue was provided along with oral information. Memory testing indicated difficulty with memory for unrelated material. Repetition of information does not improve Sally's performance, but providing memory strategies does assist and these should be used in her classroom. In addition, during the aforementioned tests Sally was found to experience some difficulty with figure–ground understanding of auditory information. Further evaluation for a possible central auditory processing disorder should be pursued.

Sally shows good thinking skills and is able to use examiner feedback. Motor assessment indicated significant weaknesses in finger dexterity and with finger tapping speed. Particular difficulty was noted in her ability to coordinate her hands when working on a task. Sally's right hand was more affected than her left. These areas require additional assessment. Behaviorally, Sally is not showing significant difficulties, as noted by parent and teacher reports. Given that the injury is only 5 months old, some of these skills may improve with time and should be monitored

In light of these findings, the following recommendations are offered:

1. It is recommended that an occupational therapy evaluation be completed either through Sally's school or through a private clinic. Given the motor findings and the continuing concerns with balance, such an assessment can assist in providing appropriate programming for Sally. Her school

district is aware of her TBI, and it appears appropriate for the school to continue to monitor Sally's progress, particularly in mathematics.

2. As there has not been a school meeting to discuss Sally's traumatic brain injury or her areas of weakness, it is important that such a meeting be held as soon as possible. Although Sally shows remarkable recovery, some areas are problematic for her and need assistance. In addition, she is spending an inordinate amount of time on homework each night—a situation that is beginning to affect her family because of the struggles over doing the work.

3. It is recommended that Sally's teacher use visual cues paired with auditory information. Sally also needs additional time to process information, and the teacher should check with her to make sure she has grasped new concepts.

4. An audiological evaluation for possible central auditory processing disorder is recommended.

5. Memory assistance is recommended, and it is strongly recommended that her teacher break larger tasks into small steps and use repetition that involves some type of memory strategies (verbal rehearsal, chunking, etc.). Helping Sally to associate what she needs to remember with a similar concept will help. She performs much better on tasks that are in context than those that are list-like or rote. Information should be presented without additional frills, which can confuse the issue. Small print should be avoided, and, as much as possible, work requiring extensive writing should be avoided. It is also recommended that Sally be seated at the center-front of the classroom to eliminate as many distractions as possible.

6. A reevaluation of Sally's skills in 1 year's time is recommended to ascertain her progress.

Following receipt of a report of this assessment, the principal at the school Sally was attending called the neuropsychologist to set up a meeting. The meeting was attended by the principal, school nurse, school psychologist, regular education teacher, occupational/physical therapist, special education teacher for children classified as "other health impaired," and Sally's mother and father. The results of the testing were summarized. Input from Sally's teacher indicated that although she was generally working within expectations for her grade, she was in the slower group of readers and behind most of her peers in mathematics. Concern was also expressed by Sally's teacher about the attentional difficulties that were noted, as well as her tendency to raise her hand and then not remember what she was going to say. The teacher also reported that Sally appeared quite fatigued by midmorning and again in midafternoon. The school day was 6½ hours long.

The principal reported that the school had believed that Sally was fully recovered, as the hospital and her doctor had not presented any records or areas of concern. A brief summary of TBI was provided by the neuropsychologist in the context of educational needs. The meeting determined that Sally did show needs under the category of TBI, and consultation of the special education teacher with the regular education teacher was recommended. In addition, the special education teacher agreed to provide individual support in mathematics and reading comprehension as needed. Homework was to be limited to 30 minutes per night. The occupational therapist had evaluated Sally's needs and found a significant need for occupational therapy and handwriting support. In addition, an evaluation of Sally's ability to attend to several auditory stimuli at one time confirmed a diagnosis of central auditory processing disorder. Recommendations were made for adjustments in the classroom and a reduction in noise through the use of an FM amplifier.

Sally's mother requested monthly meetings with her teachers to improve communication between home and school. To the same end, Sally's teacher asked for a journal to be sent back and forth to provide information about occurrences at home and school. Finally, it was recommended that the professional staff be provided with inservice instruction on TBI.

This case illustrates a not unusual situation—a child with a fairly substantial injury who had not had a psychological or neuropsychological evaluation. Her school district was in a fairly rural area, and Sally was its only identified child with TBI. Because no medical personnel had contacted the school and the school had not obtained the records, it was assumed that Sally was fine and could resume regular class attendance following the summer break. Communication broke down between home and school. Sally's mother thought that the school minimized her daughter's difficulty, and the school believed that Sally's parents were being overprotective. Assistance was needed, not only to provide a comprehensive evaluation, but also to assist in building a bridge between the home and school. This case required ongoing input from the neuropsychologist and continuing support by the school psychologist and special education staff. The inservice session that was conducted a few weeks after the multidisciplinary team meeting provided a forum in which teachers and staff could learn the intricacies of the brain–behavior relationship. In the end, the efforts of all involved were successful in providing Sally with the necessary educational support and assisting with her adjustment and eventual coping with her injury.

The following chapter provides practical suggestions for working with children with TBI in the main academic areas as well as behaviorally. It is by no means an exhaustive menu of interventions and is not meant to be a "how to" guide. Rather, ideas are presented that able teachers are well trained to adapt to their own needs and from which they can develop new ideas.

CHAPTER 8

♦♦♦

Classroom Interventions

♦

Successful reentry into school during recovery from TBI requires the coordination of all systems in the child's life: home, school, and medical. In the past, rehabilitation has basically emphasized restoring physical functioning, to the neglect of social–emotional and behavioral recovery (National Institutes of Health, 1998). Suggestions from the National Institutes of Health include the integration of school and home throughout the recovery of the child, as well as ensuring access to needed services. Research on the efficacy of educational techniques has not been forthcoming, making it difficult to determine the success of these techniques (Michaud, 1995). Yet it has been determined that children and adolescents with TBI require educational approaches that are different from the traditional curriculum, and that teachers and school psychologists are in the best position to provide such individualization and support.

The IEP or Section 504 plans set forth the goals and objectives for such interventions, but it is up to the individual teachers to implement these recommendations. This chapter offers a number of suggestions deemed helpful for the reentry of a child/adolescent into the school system, addressing each of the areas frequently found to be affected by a head injury. Ozer (1988) has provided a framework for our understanding of the most common types of deficits that interfere with school functioning and later life adjustment. These deficits include the following:

- Motor—both fine and gross motor skills
- Short-term memory and new learning
- Receptive and expressive language skills
- Problems with attention and concentration
- Visual–spatial and visual–motor deficits
- Problems with executive functions and goal setting

- Difficulty with judgment and insight
- Fatigue
- Emotional difficulties, including depression and substance abuse

Each of these areas may require specific interventions for success in the classroom. Interventions for some areas, such as fatigue, are relatively simple. For children who become fatigued after a shorter than expected amount of time, it is fairly easy to provide a nap or a time away from stimulation. Difficulties with gross and fine motor skills can be assisted through technology, physical modifications, and support. In my experience, children with gross motor deficits that are obvious handicaps are more readily provided understanding of their disabilities than children who "look normal." It is important to remember that most children who reenter the school system are generally in the later stages of recovery, and issues such as stamina, attention, severe language deficits, and severe behavioral disturbances are not as much in the forefront. Difficulties in these areas frequently remain, but children at this stage may fit into the classroom more readily (Ylvisaker, 1985). Program goals must emphasize the child's strengths as well as his/her weaknesses and should evaluate the more subtle aspects of the child's disability.

GENERAL PROGRAMMING CONSIDERATIONS

Cohen (1996) suggests that the teacher recognize the continuum of skills required for successful learning. As tasks move from concrete to abstract, a child with TBI may have difficulty in understanding cause–effect relationships and in problem solving. Moreover, the child's ability to expand ideas beyond the simple may be affected, which may result in difficulty in understanding a main idea amid many details. The most problematic area can be the application of what is newly learned to that previously learned. Such generalization can make it difficult for the child to profit from new learning, as she/he is unable to fit this new knowledge into an existing framework. Thus, new skills must be evaluated as to mastery and compensatory strategies taught for those not mastered. In addition, it is suggested that teachers determine whether the child requires reteaching of previously learned skills or whether these skills should be replaced by compensatory techniques. Thus, Cohen suggests that before proceeding with content, teachers may need to reteach the underlying skills that were automatic prior to the accident.

An initial step is to perform a task analysis to determine which skills remain and which are now missing. This analysis allows the teacher to determine *how* the child solves a problem as well as *what* he/she accomplishes. For example, a child I evaluated had difficulty in reading single words and her phonetic decoding ability appeared to be significantly affected by her head injury. However, she was able to read passages and answer questions fairly well on a standardized reading test. When her performance was evaluated, it became clear that she was misreading several of the words of the passage, while at the same time understanding the context and thus being able to successfully answer the questions. When she was asked to read a longer passage with many more details, she experienced significant difficulty with comprehension. The task itself lent to her successful comprehension and provided a window into a strategy for teaching.

A finding for children with TBI that has been replicated is the need for additional time for learning and processing of material (Mercer & Mercer, 1989). Additional practice time must also be provided in order for the child to build on previously learned skills and to retain what is being taught. Many of us wish to jump in and try to fix all of the child's difficulties at one time (Cohen, 1996). Research indicates that a more successful approach is to prioritize the necessary steps in learning and to focus on these essential skills. The shotgun approach, trying to do everything at one time, only frustrates the teacher and the child and increases the emotional upset experienced when the child sees his/her level of competency to be lower than it was before the accident (Bos & Vaughn, 1988).

It is particularly important for curricular decisions to be made for the individual child—trying to fit the child into an existing curriculum generally causes frustration and failure. Task analysis can assist in determining the steps needed for the child to master a prioritized skill. Books such as Shapiro's (1996) *Academic Skills Problems* can assist in setting up an appropriate task analysis.

Given that many children with TBI experience some difficulty with attention, it is helpful to focus the child's attention on the important parts of a lesson. Providing explicit instruction about what is important to remember as opposed to what is not can assist the child in retaining the primary points. Children with TBI can experience significant problems in differentiating relevant from irrelevant detail and may become overwhelmed when too many demands are placed on them at one time. Thus, explicit instruction such as "This is important to remember" can assist them in learning and in developing a compensating technique. I use this strategy when teaching an overview course for undergraduates, and it has been reported to be very helpful. To many undergraduates, everything in a book appears to be important, so they may underline almost an entire text—not a very helpful technique for studying. Compound this problem several-fold for a child with TBI, and recognize that it is important for the teacher to emphasize priorities and to help the child organize the myriad of details encountered throughout the school day.

Cohen (1996) suggests that teachers focus the child's attention by using verbal cues that request the child *to organize, to be flexible, or to initiate tasks.* All of these cues signal to the child that these are important skills that must be remembered. Cohen goes on to suggest that these key words be used throughout the child's school day and by all of the child's teachers to further emphasize the need for the child to think operationally about what he/she is learning and not just about content. Additional cue words and phrases include the following:

- Focus
- Remember
- Evaluate
- Plan
- Apply
- How does it work?
- What did you do to solve the problem?

In addition to using cue words, it is helpful to provide real-life experiences in which to apply the new learning. Such practical learning experiences provide opportunities for the child to apply the learning and, therefore, to practice new skills directly after instruction. Transfer of learning is a particularly difficult area for many children, but particularly for children with TBI, and linkage of this kind can assist the child in such generalization. The ability of the child to apply learning can be enhanced through active learning and hands-on learning. Demonstration of learning, as well as talking through the process of problem solving, can assist the child in developing compensatory strategies. An awareness that there is more than one way to solve a problem can also assist the child in developing flexibility of thought and in bolstering self-esteem upon success (Cohen, 1991; Prigatano, 2000).

With hands-on learning also comes the ability to use a multisensory approach, using several input channels at one time to enhance the child's learning. Such an approach has been found to be very helpful for children with TBI as well as for those with other types of learning disabilities (Savage & Wolcott, 1988; Ylvisaker, 1985). By allowing a child to complete a task beyond the usual paper and pencil method, a teacher can provide an opportunity for the child to explore knowledge through various mediums and enhance the child's willingness to try new activities. As the child solves a problem, the teacher can scaffold the learning so that the child takes on ever more responsibility within a safe learning environment (Vygotsky, 1993) In this manner, the child can attempt tasks that may initially seem too difficult. Through modeling, the teacher can verbalize and demonstrate how tasks are broken down and how to plan and organize a task that may at first seem overwhelming.

Consistent with the need to break down cognitive tasks into their component parts, behavior and social expectations also require such treatment. Plain discussion of expectations is helpful for many children with special needs, and particularly for those with TBI. Outlining expectations can provide support for the child and clarify any confusion about the teacher's expectations (Cohen et al., 1985). Unfortunately, many teachers believe that once stated, the rules are understood and enforcement should not engender any confusion. Work with children with TBI (as well as those with ADHD) indicates just the opposite; often, when asked why he/she has lost points or has been given detention, the child will honestly reply, "But I didn't do anything wrong." In one case, a child experienced significant difficulty recalling a teacher's instructions, particularly when more than one direction was given at a time—a frequent occurrence in the classroom. She asked her seatmate what the directions were and was told by the teacher to stop talking. In this situation, the child was hesitant to tell the teacher that she did not understand and thus lost points toward a reward. When this difficulty continued over time, the teacher was experienced enough to question why the child was talking out of turn, particularly just before independent seatwork. A task analysis indicated the difficulty with understanding multiple directions, and an intervention was introduced to provide additional support.

In summary, general considerations must be addressed in teaching children with TBI, prior to specific interventions. General skills lay the foundation for the development of more specific skills and for learning the compensatory techniques that allow the child to benefit from general instruction.

SPECIFIC INTERVENTIONS

Specific interventions for deficits in attention, memory, social skills, and cognitive processing ability are discussed in the following sections with an eye to the development of learning strategies. These strategies emphasize the development of independence for learning and the ability to generalize what has been learned to a new situation. The overall goal, of course, is to move the child from reliance on special education and services to attendance in the regular classroom for as much of the day as possible.

Attention

As discussed in Chapter 3, attention and concentration difficulties are frequently seen in children with TBI. Because such problems can negatively affect new learning, it is particularly important for the teacher to provide additional support in these areas. Specific interventions that have been adapted from Braswell and Bloomquist (1991) include making changes in the environment, in worksheet and lesson presentation, and in behavioral management. Environmental considerations include priority seating for the child—children who sit where the teacher is generally located improve in attention. For many children this may mean seating at the center-front of the classroom. For others, whose teachers move about the room, it is particularly important that an effort be made to establish eye or physical contact to keep the child on task. Reducing extraneous distractions is also important, and seating away from a window may be helpful. Possibly most helpful is to seat the child next to peers who have adequate attentional skills. In my experience, it often happens that a child with poor attentional ability is seated in the back of the room with other children who have similar problems. Although some classroom environments require the use of tables grouped in sets of four, the best seating for children with attentional problems may be an arrangement whereby seats are placed in rows.

Lesson presentation is another area in which adaptations can be very helpful. A teacher can assist older students by providing an outline of a lesson and a vocabulary sheet. These advanced organizers can help them to prepare for the lesson. Many children with TBI tend to have difficulty with slow processing time, and such outlines can allow a child to keep up with the lesson and to be aware of what is coming next, and may possibly allow time for questioning on a particular point. Younger children with TBI require lessons that are varied and brief. Instructions should be clearly provided, and it is helpful to have a list of tasks that must be accomplished each day written on the board. Cooperative learning activities may be most helpful for children and adolescents with TBI, in that they are not required to complete an entire task alone. Providing learning stations may add variety to the lesson presentation. Learning stations that allow for self-correction have been found to be helpful for children with ADHD and likely will assist those with TBI (Braswell & Bloomquist, 1991). Colored chalk can be used to discriminate between various ideas, and overheads and other visual aids can also be helpful in presentations.

Worksheets can be adapted for children with TBI through the use of larger type and good contrast between print and background. The use of dittos should be discouraged, as the print can easily blend into the background. It is best to avoid clutter on a page and to keep the format simple. Encountering several tasks on a single page can be overwhelming for a child with TBI. Rather than attempt to put everything on one page, it is far better to provide additional pages with one type of task on each. Well-planned worksheets can help a child with the organization of his/her work and can add to the feeling of accomplishment as each page is completed. Highlighting key directions and vocabulary words can provide visual cues as to relevant versus irrelevant details.

Frequent reminders to check their work are also helpful, as many children with TBI and/or ADHD tend to have difficulty with realizing mistakes. This permits the teacher to assist the child in checking the work, and provides a model for the development of executive functions. A frequently used strategy for successful test taking is to allow the child/adolescent to take a test orally; this strategy is particularly helpful when basic reading skills are unreliable. Moreover, it is helpful to provide practice tests to allow the child to learn *how* to take tests.

Following the standards of behavior can be problematic for children with TBI, and it is a particularly good idea for the teacher to make sure that rules are not only clear but also posted in a visible area. Charting behavior can be quite helpful for children with TBI. As mentioned earlier, these children have difficulty in their ability to self-monitor their skills. Charting provides a reminder of what is problematic for the child, as well as what can be helpful, and a measure of his/her progress. Another easily made modification can assist the child in developing his/her ability to set priorities. By allowing the child a choice in what he/she does first and then second, the child is provided an opportunity to evaluate the progress made and to anticipate what needs to be completed within the time allotted. It is very helpful for a child, and particularly for an adolescent, to set both short- and long-term goals for skill learning and behavior. By analyzing the child's progress, it is possible to provide the child with support for his/her behavior and to model appropriate self-monitoring and insight behaviors.

In addition to the preceding suggestions, Harrington (1990) suggests that the child should be provided continuing reminders to focus his/her attention and then be rewarded when he/she has done so. In addition, it is important that assignments be relevant to the task at hand, that rote work and drill be kept to a minimum, and that fatigue be carefully monitored. Moreover, any medication the child is taking should be monitored for efficacy, and close contact between home and school should be maintained. Additional suggestions can be found in Barkley's (2000) *Taking Charge of ADHD*.

Mateer and colleagues (1996) correctly point out that our knowledge of working with attentional disorders is derived from the literature on adult head injury. Additional information is provided in the literature on ADHD. The application of these works to children with TBI needs further study. Mateer and colleagues suggest that speed of information processing is related to attention as a limiting factor; that is, when the child is unable to process information at a usual pace, attention becomes scattered and performance is negatively affected. Such difficulties may lead to problems with divided attention, which results from the ability to focus on more than one task at a time. For example, when driving a car most people can talk to another person or listen to the radio with only a small decrement in performance. At this point the task is automatic. However, if you are attempting to drive in a downpour, the task becomes more cognitively driven and you find it difficult to divide your attention between the main task and the accompanying distractions. For the child with TBI most work may be likened to your driving in a downpour—full attention must be paid to the task at hand, and any other requirements either cause poor performance or are not processed.

The preceding suggestions include modifications to the environment and to teaching behavior. Additional work has indicated that direct retraining may also be helpful for children with TBI. This literature is based mainly on studies of adults with TBI. There is some emerging evidence in regard to direct retraining and ADHD, but further study is needed (Semrud-Clikeman et al., 1999). Retraining programs stress repeated opportunities to practice a variety of attention skills. The Attention Process Training (APT) program (Sohlberg & Mateer, 1987) provides hierarchically organized tasks based on a model of attention that is multidimensional, including focused attention, sustained attention, selective attention, alternating attention, and divided attention (Sohlberg & Mateer, 1989a).

Focused attention involves the ability to attend to specific input. In the early stages of TBI focused attention may be problematic, but these difficulties resolve with recovery. Sustained attention requires the ability to pay attention to a continuous and repetitive activity. Continuous performance tests tap this type of attention. It is usually the case that children with difficulty with sustained attention can focus on a task for only a short period of time or that their attentional skills are inconsistent, depending on the intrinsic interest of the task (video games). Mateer and colleagues (1996) suggest that working memory skills (the ability to hold more than one piece of information in mind at a time) constitute a higher cognitive level of sustained attention. Selective attention requires the ability to maintain attention to task when distracting information is present. Children with TBI often have difficulty in working on tasks in a noisy or busy environment. Alternating attention requires the ability to shift one's focus during a task— for example, the ability to listen to a lecture and take notes.

The APT program includes a number of tasks that gradually increase in difficulty to improve the child's attentional capacity in the five attention areas. The APT requires additional training and small-group or individual administration. Emerging evidence for improvement in attentional capacity for children with ADHD has been found in two studies. Williams (1989) studied six children with ADHD using the APT materials. Significant improvements were found on the training tasks, with a trend toward improvement in academic skills. Semrud-Clikeman and colleagues (1999) studied children who were identified by regular classroom teachers as having problems with work completion and attention. These children were not, for the most part, on medication and were not in special education. The APT materials were used over an 18-week period, with improvement noted on visual and auditory attention tasks and in homework completion.

APT has also been applied to six children with TBI, with significant gains found on measures of attention and timed mathematics activities (Thomson, 1995). Additional support for the use of APT with children with TBI comes from a case study of two children with severe TBI presented by Thomson and Kerns (in press). The tasks were modified for the severe difficulties of these children and are presently being studied for outcome efficacy.

Although the APT materials are promising, more research is needed to improve their application and ease of use. It appears that the most fruitful program would incorporate environmental changes as well as neuropsychological changes for these children. The environmental modifications are generally within the training experience of most teachers and are readily implemented with little cost. It is recommended that both accommodations be considered, depending on the children's needs.

Memory

Difficulties with memory and new learning are the most frequent sequelae of TBI (Telzrow, 1987). A problem in this area can affect the child's ability to profit from instruction as well as his/her emotional and social adjustment. In addition, memory difficulties can increase anxiety as the child/adolescent worries about whether he/she will recall learned information on another occasion (Wilson & Moffat, 1984). Sohlberg and Mateer (1987) suggest that although memory deficits cannot be remediated, the child can be taught strategies to assist memory skills. These compensations can involve external (computers, etc.) or internal strategies (Mateer et al., 1996).

Internal Memory Strategies

Internal memory strategies that have been found helpful include chunking of information, association learning, and mnemonic strategies. Chunking of information requires the child to reduce the information to be learned into smaller portions that are related to each other. For example, learning a Social Security number can be chunked into three segments and then rehearsed. Association learning requires the child to relate the new learning to something that has already been learned. The child is thus assisted in developing a framework to draw upon when required to retrieve the information.

Mnemonic techniques include the recall of information based on associations. For example, the initial letters of the phrase "every good boy does fine" allow one to recall the names of the notes on a music staff. Sohlberg and Mateer (1989a) suggest a similar strategy for recalling the colors of the rainbow—"Roy G. Biv" (red, orange, yellow, green, blue, indigo, and violet). Involving the child in developing such a memory strategy can also help him/her to apply the strategy independently. Another mnemonic technique is to use visual or sensory associations. Associating a distinctive facial feature with a name helps many of us to recall a person the next time we see him/her. Relating an item to be remembered with a past experience can also aid in remembering it.

Still another strategy to improve recall is to rehearse the new information, reciting it out loud. For example, needing to recall a telephone number, we may repeat it several times until we dial it. Such rehearsal can aid children in recalling important information. It has also been found that stressing the importance of remembering information (e.g., having the child state, "I must remember this") can assist in recall. Writing the material to be remembered also appears to strengthen the memory trace (Cohen, 1996). Paring down the information into its important parts is helpful as well—eliminate the frills and emphasize the essential details.

For some tasks, it is important to recall certain information. The use of recognition cues may be sufficient, rather than a reliance on rote memory. Providing advanced organizers (e.g., an outline) for a lesson can help the child to attend to the material without having to focus on various items for recall. Preparing the child in advance for what is to be learned appears to assist in retention of the material (Woolfolk, 2001). In addition, the use of extensive repetition can assist in improving the memory trace. This type of repetition can most readily be accomplished with computer programs designed to improve memory skills. Such programs are available through education suppliers and the Cambridge Laboratory (1-800-637-0047).

External Aids

External aids are available through computer outlets and educational stores. Computerized devices such as Palm Pilots, organizers, and calendars provide support for recalling details that are important but not necessary to memorize. These devices can be used to store specific experiences, lists of things that have to be done, and important information. Such aids can be devised specifically for the persons using them.

Although these devices are a great addition to the resources used in working with children and adolescents, the child/adolescent must be trained in their use and encouraged to use them. It is important for the teacher to model their use and to provide practice based on everyday life.

However, a strategy must not be so cumbersome that it interferes with functioning. For example, a client's teacher was very well intentioned and devised a system to assist him in remembering his materials and books. Each subject was assigned a folder of a different color matched to a notebook of the same color—science, red; social studies, blue; English, green. Although this system may work for well-organized students, for my client it became increasingly confusing. He could not remember what color matched which course and continually brought the wrong folder and notebook to class. The system was so fraught with memory difficulties that it did not assist this student and further complicated his life. We solved the problem by using one organizer that was divided into classes and required him to remember only one item.

Teaching the use of such external aids does not come naturally and requires motivation on the part of the student and teacher. Sohlberg and Mateer (1989b) suggest a three-stage behavioral program for teaching the use of external aids. First, a task analysis and behavioral observations pinpoint when and how a particular external aid may be used. At this stage the child is trained in how to use the aid. Second, the child is trained in when to use the aid, and, finally, he/she is taught how to apply the training to the everyday world. This system was found to be effective in a case study, improving the child's ability to complete tasks appropriately and on time (Kerns et al., 1993).

The use of such memory devices has not been fully studied, and additional work is needed in this area. In any case, it is important to provide training and practice in the use of these systems as well as frequent review about their application. These developments are exciting, and it is important to explore the use of such technology to assist the child in compensating. A limitation may be the affordability of such devices, and many schools are reluctant to provide this equipment. If it is believed that such technology is necessary, the child should be referred for an assistive technology evaluation.

Executive Functions

Problem-solving skills constitute one of the areas most in need of intervention and one of the most difficult. Training the child to think independently, to be cognitively flexible enough to generalize solutions, and to transfer learning can be challenging tasks in teaching children with TBI or other disabilities. Executive functioning is an important skill throughout life, as it allows a person to change a problem-solving set depending on the situation at hand. Thus, it is important to assist the child in developing the appropriate skills in order to plan, organize, prioritize, and apply various strategies.

One way to assist in this area is to provide open-ended questions that encourage the child to think for him/herself and to evaluate the solution that is applied. For children with memory difficulties, the use of multiple-choice questions may be most appropriate, as they assist in the retrieval of the information required and thus diminish the memory requirement (Cohen, 1996).

A main component of executive functioning is the ability to self-monitor. This skill is particularly important for a child with TBI, in order to avoid repeating mistakes and to learn from new experiences. Self-monitoring includes the ability to recognize when you are feeling overwhelmed or when you need help. Many children and adolescents with TBI are reluctant to ask, and it is important to assist them when they show signs of needing help. The child's ability to evaluate his/her performance is essential to self-monitoring. The use of charts and feedback on performance has been found to aid skill development in self-monitoring (Semrud-Clikeman et al., 1999).

Teachers, both regular and special education, may wish to use charts as visual aids to assist the child in assessing his/her performance and developing strategies to improve performance. Semrud-Clikeman and colleagues (1999) successfully used charts and feedback to encourage children with attention and work completion problems to evaluate their progress and reassess the problem-solving skills being used. For example, the children were repeatedly tested on materials that required sustained attention and accurate completion. If a child worked too quickly, accuracy declined; if the child was very slow, the time allotted for the task was not sufficient. Each child was encouraged to try different solutions to a problem. When too much speed was used at the sacrifice of accuracy, this solution was evaluated by the child and the examiner and adjusted accordingly. Such training can be used in both regular and special education settings. The children were also encouraged to predict how they would do on a task, and these predictions were then evaluated upon completion.

The development of goals is an integral part of executive functioning skills. Programs in cognitive–behavioral therapy can be quite helpful, particularly in developing self-monitoring skills (Bloomquist & Braswell, 1991; Kendall & Braswell, 1993). These programs can also be helpful in working with impulsive behavior.

For the use of goals and performance criteria to be helpful, frequent review is necessary, preferably on an individual basis. The use of metacognitive strategies to assist in goal setting requires the child be aware of what is to be learned. Attention is a precursor for such awareness, and the teacher must be confident that the child understands what is expected of him/her. Once the requirement is understood, the application of cognitive strategies can be quite helpful. These strategies can include the following:

- A structured environment with set expectations
- Rehearsal of what is expected of the child (First, I need to do x, and then I need to do y)
- Setting priorities as to what has to be done first, second, and so on
- Teaching brainstorming procedures
  - Identify the problem
  - Obtain information about the problem
  - Generate alternative solutions; determine pros and cons
  - Select the solution
  - Make a plan for application of the solution
  - Evaluate the solution
- Frequent feedback as to performance on the tasks
- Reevaluation of the strategies used if success is not achieved
- Frequent meetings between teacher and student
- Modeling of appropriate problem-solving skills
- Providing practice in the child's self-evaluation of his/her skills

Planning deficits are also frequently found in children with TBI or other disabilities. Such deficits are found particularly when there is damage to the frontal lobes. Planning deficits can confound many of the teaching strategies outlined earlier. The child may be attempting to organize his/her thinking but is unable to carry through with the plan because of difficulty in prioritizing the material. An example of an organization plan is provided in Table 8.1. This plan was adapted from Braswell and Bloomquist (1991). Additional suggestions are also available through Canter and Carroll's *Helping Children at Home and School* (1998).

Academics

Although children with TBI can profit from the same types of interventions frequently used for children with learning disabilities, it is particularly relevant for the teacher to recall that a child's rate of information processing may differ from that of other children his/her age. Such differential processing may interfere with the child's ability to profit from instruction and cause problems in interpreting what has been said. The attentional requirements for listening to a lecture while taking notes may be too great for children with TBI, and it is important that additional support be provided as necessary, such as engaging peer notetakers or allowing a child to tape-record a lesson. It cannot be overemphasized that if the child is not able to input information, the amount of retention can be nil—not because of learning problems but because of input difficulty. Thus, Savage and Wolcott (1988) suggest that verbal material be presented in at a slower

TABLE 8.1. General Strategies for Organization

These strategies should not be implemented all at once. Give the child, Sam, just one strategy at a time and, when he is comfortable with it, add another. The goal is for Sam to internalize these strategies and be able to use them *on his own*, not just when he is reminded to do so by others. It may also be helpful for a reward system to be implemented at home and/or at school to help reinforce and build in these strategies.

At home
a. Sam should be encouraged to use just *one* notebook/organizing system (e.g., Mead's Trapper/Keeper) for *all* his classes (instead of using different notebooks for different classes).
b. Daily homework assignments should be prioritized and checked off when they are completed. Initially he will need help and guidance both at home and at school in using this system, but should gradually learn to do so on his own.
c. Parents can help Sam at home by keeping his school-related materials in one place (e.g., on a desk or in a special study area). Easy-to-follow rules and routines regarding when and where homework is to be done may also be helpful. At night, Sam can be encouraged to gather all his school materials and leave them in a backpack by the door.
d. Schedule time each week for Sam to go through his desk, backpack, and notebooks to remove papers and items that are no longer needed. School papers should be filed in a binder that has a section for each subject.
e. A monthly calendar can be used to list due dates for long-term projects, papers, and reports.

At school
a. Sam's school may consider providing him with a second set of textbooks to keep at home if he has difficulty remembering to take books home with him.
b. Sam should be helped to write down his assignments for each class in his Assignment Book and to check off each task when he has completed it.
c. Sam will likely need additional assistance in getting started with large, multistep tasks and prioritizing what to do. Help him by giving him a starting point and asking him what to do next. When he is finished with one or two steps, ask him to identify the next step.

---

pace with repetition provided as necessary. In addition, it is recommended that, as much as possible, verbal information be paired with a visual clue.

Reading

Reading is a particularly important skill that TBI can affect significantly. Generally, if the child has mastered the mechanics prior to the injury, the difficulty may lie in comprehension of the material. If the mechanics have not been mastered before the injury, specific programs, such as the Lindamood (Lindamood & Lindamood, 1998) or FastForWord (Tallal et al., 1996) program may be appropriate for the development of basic reading skills. Rosner and colleagues (1981) provide a program that encourages the development of auditory analysis of spoken language, which has been found helpful in remediation for children with learning disabilities.

Sight Word Vocabulary

Word recognition is particularly important for the child with learning problems. Deshler and colleagues (1984) designed a program to help students quickly identify unknown words in their reading material, through a seven-step problem-solving procedure to decode words. Using the acronym DISSECT, students learn to read multisyllable words:

D   Discover the context
I   Isolate the prefix
S   Separate the suffix
S   Say the stem
E   Examine the stem
C   Check with someone
T   Try the dictionary

For younger children sight word recognition is particularly important, and automatization of the process is necessary for reading comprehension. A child who struggles over the reading of single words will often not understand what has been read. Thus, it is important for the decoding process to become automatized. Younger children can profit from direct teacher instruction in basic reading skills that are often taken for granted—for example, examining the cover of a book and predicting, from the title, what the book is about. Having the teacher read aloud can model reading, provide an exercise in attention to task, and allow for a discussion of what has been read. To increase sight word vocabulary, the child can read along while listening to a taped reading by the teacher of the same material. In this way, the child learns the words within a context.

The use of a matching approach, in which a word is initially presented with a pictorial representation, also facilitates sight word recognition. This approach allows children to recognize a word in context or in isolation (as explained in Berninger et al., 1997). Teachers can use the following steps:

1. The word is presented with a picture on a flash card. For example, the teacher introduces the word by stating, "This is a car."
2. Next, more than one picture card is presented to students.
3. This step is similar to step 2, but the pictures are not presented with

the words. The teacher introduces the activity by asking, "Which is the car?" "Which is the pan?"

4. At this step the teacher asks students to read words presented on cards without pictures. The teacher introduces the activity by asking, "What is this word?" At each of the preceding levels, the teacher may provide students with printed cards of the introduced vocabulary. The students can then use them to form sentences or stories.

5. In this final step, the teacher asks students to read in sentences by putting the words on cards together. There are two considerations involved in presenting sentences: (a) Use language structures that are within children's repertoire, and (b) embed new words in the middle or at the ends of the sentences to provide more semantic and syntactic information.

In addition, the learning of new words can be aided by using a color-coded system. Words can be color-coded as whole words, as parts of words, or as desired sounds, such as initial consonant sounds and various vowel sound combinations. These interventions have been found helpful in the Lindamood system. Games of Concentration, Scrabble, Scattergories, and Bingo can also be used to build sight words. In addition, it is important to create a classroom (and home) environment that encourages and values reading. Teachers (and parents) who model not only the purpose of reading, but also a love for reading, have been found to have children who are more open to the reading process (Woolfolk, 2001).

Reading Comprehension

Instruction in self-questioning attempts to show students how to draw meaningful information from text and how to monitor their comprehension of text material. In this process students are encouraged to generate questions about the important parts of the text, such as, What is the main idea in the paragraph? What are the supporting details? In addition, the students can be taught to generate questions that help them self-monitor comprehension: Do I understand the material read? Do I know the main idea? Is there anything I don't understand in this paragraph? How does it relate to my life? Similarly, teachers can model for students how to ask questions pertaining to story structure elements: Who are the main characters in the story? What is the aim of the story?

Story mapping has also been found helpful in improving comprehension. This technique assists the child in mapping out the most important aspects of the story. It is similar to the SQ4R technique frequently used for study skills remediation (Woolfolk, 2001). SQ4R asks the child to do the following:

- Survey the material—read the title and the headings.
- Question—read the questions at the end of the chapter.
- Read—read the chapter.
- Recite—after reading the chapter, recite the main points.
- Review—review the chapter and the questions.
- Reread—read the chapter again.

A story map and the following set of questions are used to teach story mapping:

1. Where did the story take place?
2. When did this story take place?
3. Who were the main characters in the story?
4. Were there any other important characters in the story? Who?
5. What was the problem in the story?

The use of such techniques has been found to improve not only reading comprehension but also study skills in children up to college age who have difficulties in learning (Weinstein, 1994). The use of structure further assists children with TBI in that it allows for the organization of material to be learned and provides a framework for future learning.

Writing

Writing skills are also frequently affected by TBI; a child may have difficulty with both the writing mechanics themselves and the organization of ideas to be written. Berninger (1998) has developed a program that provides assistance in organizing ideas and thoughts and support in the writing process.

In many cases the difficulty for the child with TBI may lie in the organization of ideas, for which the preceding suggestions are helpful. The most important task is to determine where the breakdown in writing occurs. The use of standardized tests can be helpful, but supplementing these materials with informal measures is also important. An assessment of the child's writing performance on daily tasks can assist in the necessary analysis of the child's skills. Providing a model for the child of what should be said in his/her writing can also be helpful. The story mapping technique discussed earlier can be readily applied to the writing process as a way of organizing the material to be written.

Richards (1998) suggests an eight-step process in teaching writing skills, which she entitles POWER (plan, organize thoughts and ideas, write, edit, revise):

- Encourage the child to think about ideas for his/her writing and talk through each of the ideas.
- Use a mind map to help organize the ideas—put the main idea in a center circle and connect the supporting ideas to the center.

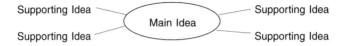

- Make a list of words that the child is unsure of spelling.
- Write a draft of the paper with the focus on ideas, not sentence structure.
- Proofread—use the grammar and spell checker on a word processor.
- Revise.
- Proofread again.
- Print out the final product.

Richards (1998) also suggests that it is quite important to evaluate the speed of the writing to determine whether there are problems in the formulation of ideas, in the organization of ideas, or in the writing process itself. If the mechanical process of writing is the problem, then it is important to determine whether assistive technology is required. Teaching a child keyboarding can be particularly important when a motor difficulty is impairing the writing process. For other tasks, it may be appropriate for the child to tape-record what is to be written. With newer computer technology, the child can speak into the computer, which then provides a written output of the material.

For handwriting improvement, it is important for the child to be corrected in letter formation and to be provided with practice so that correct letter formation can be automatized and writing can become fluent. Richards (1998) suggests that air writing large letters can help the child to develop more efficient motor traces of writing and can reinforce the correct formation of letters. She also maintains that these skills must be practiced until they are automatized before children can be expected to use them in writing their ideas.

Mathematics

Skills in mathematics can be affected by difficulties in spatial orientation, memory for mathematics facts, and difficulties with mathematics reasoning skills. It is particularly important to isolate the area of difficulty in mathematics, just as in reading. Unfortunately, there is less empirical research into the various techniques that can be helpful for mathematics instruction.

If a child is asked to solve 56 – 4 and the child answers 16, it is likely that the difficulty lies in the aligning of the numbers. In this case, the use of graph paper can assist the child in aligning columns. It is also helpful to teach the child to self-monitor his/her solutions.The child should be taught to ask him/herself, Does this make sense?

There is greater difficulty when the child is able to recall facts but cannot recall how to complete a mathematics process. Confusion of multiplication and addition can change an answer dramatically. Inability to remember fractions and decimals can also significantly interfere with learning. In this case, it is important for the child to overlearn this material and to be provided with additional practice. The use of concrete aids, such as Cuisenaire rods, can also be helpful, particularly in understanding fractions. Cuisenaire rods are color-coded for various units of 10. For instance, units of 1 are red and those representing 2 units (or $^1/_5$) are yellow. With these rods a child can build equations—5 units of yellow equal 1 blue (worth 10 units), and so on. The use of these aids can make it more readily apparent how numbers work and provide visual clues about the correctness of the responses. Number lines can also assist the child with the order of numbers and give visual cues for subtraction and addition. The use of calculators makes sense once the child understands how the numbers are obtained.

Word problems are a frequent stumbling block for many children. For the child with TBI, word problems may be even more difficult, as they require memory of processes as well as interpretation of what is being asked. Direct teaching of key words is essential. For example, the words "How much altogether?" mean "You are to add the numbers." Listing key words on a master paper to which the child can refer can also be helpful.

For adolescents, algebra and geometry can be particularly intimidating. It is important that the teacher conduct a thorough task analysis to determine where the breakdown in skills lies. For example, lack of memory for theorems in geometry can significantly affect the child's performance (Rosen & Gerring, 1986). A chart listing the major theorems can be helpful to any adolescent, but particularly for an adolescent with TBI. Algebraic solutions generally follow set patterns, and a chart providing samples of the various kinds of equations and their solutions can also be helpful. Generally, the breakdown is in the *process* of the task, and anything that reduces the memory requirement can help these children.

Social and Behavioral Difficulties

Difficulties in the social and behavioral areas in children and adolescents with TBI can be the most difficult with which to work (Prigatano, 1985). Plans to deal with these concerns must be included in an IEP and should provide assistance within the school environment and support for the family (Harrington,

1990). With more severe brain damage, the likelihood of behavioral and social difficulties increases (Wood, 1987), with frontal lobe damage likely accounting for the most severe behavioral disturbances (Mapou, 1992).

Kehle and colleagues (1996) report that although behavioral difficulties can significantly limit the academic and social success of students with TBI, there is little empirical evidence that one intervention strategy is more effective than another. Individual therapy, peer support groups, and communication classes may be helpful for these children and provide additional support for parents. In addition, behavioral management techniques can be quite helpful in assisting with the child's behavior. These techniques must provide positive reinforcement as well as consequences for behavior. Rules and expectations should be clearly spelled out for the child/adolescent, along with the consequences, both positive and negative. Helping the child with insight into his/her strengths and weaknesses is important, as is assisting the child in evaluating his/her own behavior (Harrington, 1990). Such insight can allow for constructive feedback and correction. Kehle and colleagues recommend that the type of intervention be selected on the basis of the child's strengths and weaknesses. For example, a student with significant difficulty with insight is not likely to benefit from insight-based (or talk) therapy (Semrud-Clikeman, 1995).

Harrington (1990) also suggests that the environment be evaluated as to the possibility of its including too much stimulation and thus negatively affecting the child's ability to cope with the demands of the classroom. Deficits in executive functioning can affect behavior significantly, particularly when it comes to solving problems. Difficulty with motivation can also be problematic and is frequently associated with TBI (Mapou, 1992). A child's awareness of poor progress and continuing frustration can be related to depression and low self-esteem, thus interfering with future progress (Kehle et al., 1996).

Aggression and noncompliance have been found to be among the more common, and problematic, difficulties in children with TBI (Kehle et al., 1986; Wood, 1987). Aggression can include impulsive behavior and/or overreaction to environmental input. Wood (1987) reports that the impulsive type of aggression can lead to violent behavior. It is important to establish clear consequences for impulsive behavior and to provide structure to avoid confrontations. For overreaction to environmental input, the solution is to provide supports within the environment to assist the child with his/her reaction and to decrease the stimulation.

Noncompliant behavior can be related to difficulty in understanding what is expected and may be a learned response to such frustration (Rhode et al., 1993). Teachers generally use reprimands in an attempt to deal with noncompliance and aggression, giving a reprimand as frequently as every 2 minutes in elementary and middle school to correct behavior (Reavis et al., 1993). Children with disabilities, particularly those with deficits in cognitive and/or social skills, are more likely to receive such reprimands (Kehle et al., 1996). As such, the frequent use of reprimands can be generally counterproductive and result in a negative teacher–child relationship. It is recommended that when a reprimand is used, it should be in statement form and connected to what is expected of the child and the consequences that will follow if a request is not honored (Reavis et al., 1993).

The use of praise in conjunction with reprimands has been found to increase compliance. Unfortunately, praise statements appear to decrease with increasing grade level (Kehle et al., 1996). It has been suggested that the ratio of praise statements to reprimands should be 4 to 1 (Reavis et al., 1993). Thus, increasing praise for appropriate behavior may well improve compliance rates. However, when a reprimand is necessary, it is important that the student realize that the teacher is prepared to follow through with the consequence.

Modeling of appropriate behavior has been found to be helpful for children with TBI (Kehle et al., 1986), improving compliance and decreasing their aggression (Kehle & Gonzales, 1991). Modeling includes the use of videotaping, to show the child complying with a request, and live modeling by another child who is in compliance. In addition, emerging empirical evidence indicates that to be most effective, such modeling is best provided on separate occasions over time rather than in one extended session (Dempster, 1988). Kehle and colleagues (1996) illustrated the use of this technique with a young girl who had compliance difficulties. She was videotaped complying with instructions. She then viewed the tape, being instructed to stop the tape each time she observed herself responding appropriately to the teacher's instruction. She was rewarded for these observed responses and her actual classroom level of compliance, which was charted. Increases were found in the girl's compliance, in her completion of work required, and in peer expectations of her behavior.

Consequences, ranging from time-outs to overcorrection, can also be helpful. A time-out is appropriate when the child finds the classroom environment reinforcing but does not work as well when the classroom is viewed as punitive. Overcorrection can assist in teaching appropriate behaviors; it requires the child to comply with instruction and provides practice in the required behavior. Kehle and colleagues (1996) caution that this type of intervention can be embarrassing to the student and should be used with this concern in mind.

PHARMACOTHERAPY

Medications may also be used as interventions for difficulties in attention and mood disorders. For some children with TBI, seizures co-occur with problems in attention, and medications must be carefully monitored. Stimulants may reduce the threshold for seizure activity, and although helpful, must be frequently evaluated (Semrud-Clikeman & Wical, 1999). Wilens (1999) provides an excellent guide to frequently used psychiatric medication.

Cope (1987) has suggested that medications should be used after behavioral and environmental modifications have proved unsuccessful. Cautious use of medications can assist the child, but overuse can be damaging. It is important to establish a baseline for behavior prior to medication so as to be able to evaluate the effectiveness of the intervention (Cope, 1987). It is well known that just giving the medication often produces improvement—a result known as the "placebo effect" (Barkley, 1998).

Attention

The most common medications used for attention include methylphenidate (Ritalin) and Adderall. Both of these medications are short-acting and leave the body in a matter of hours. They have been found to be quite effective with children with ADHD, with improvement found in attention, impulse control, and inhibition. Improvement following medication has not been found in the area of academics, as these skills must be taught directly (Barkley, 1998). Side effects of these medications include weight loss, sleep disturbances, headaches and/or stomachaches that disappear with time, and irritability once the medication begins to wear off (also called a rebound effect). Thus, it is generally recommended that children taking these medications eat prior to being given a dose and that a dose is not given within 4 hours of bedtime. These medications have also been associated with the development of tics, which may or may not be precursors to Tourette syndrome. Therefore, any tics that are noted should be monitored carefully by the child's physician.

Aggressive and Disruptive Behaviors

The use of medication for aggressive and violent behaviors has increased with the availability of a variety of new medications (Rose, 1988). Antiepileptic medications such as Tegretol and Depakote have been found to be useful in treating violent and aggressive behavior in children with and without TBI. At times medications generally prescribed for anxiety (clonidine) have been found helpful, as have lithium salts, a medication associated with bipolar disorder (Clark et al., 1990; Glenn, 1987). Antidepressants such as Prozac or Zoloft have been found helpful for some children, as have neuroleptics including Respiradol.

Seizures

There are several medications used in the treatment of seizure disorders, which have varying side effects. The most common include phenobarbitol, Dilantin, Tegretol, and Depakote. Phenobarbital, used particularly with younger children, is associated with drowsiness and attentional difficulty. Some research has implicated this medication with side effects manifested in cognitive deficits (Aldenkamp, 1995). Such cognitive deficits are of concern particularly for children with TBI, as they already have difficulties in attention and learning skills. Dilantin, Tegretol, and Depakote are also frequently prescribed, having fewer cognitive side effects than phenobarbitol.

Children with seizure disorders appear to be more susceptible to attentional deficits, and those with TBI and seizure disorder appear to be at highest risk. Research into the effect of seizure medication on attention has indicated some improvement when methylphenidate is also administered. However, this improvement was below that of children with ADHD on methylphenidate (Semrud-Clikeman & Wical, 1999).

For some children, a number of antiepileptic medications are used. These children appear to have a more severe form of seizure disorder. The use of multiple medications to control seizures appears to be related to poor academic and social performance (Aldenkamp, 1995). Thus, as more medications are added to the mix, the severity of these deficits is more intense due to side effects and the side effects are more observable. These concerns must be communicated to both the regular and special education teachers, as well as to the parents.

Mood Disorders

It is not uncommon for children with TBI to experience mood disorders. As these feelings of sadness and/or worry increase, medication may be attempted as a way to improve functioning. There are several classes of medications that can be used, and the interested reader is referred to Wilens (1999) for a full explanation of the wide array of available medications.

The most commonly utilized medications for mood disorder include selective serotonin reuptake inhibitors (SSRIs), which, because they have few side effects, are frequently prescribed for mood disorders. These medications include Prozac, Luvox, and Paxil. Zoloft and Wellbutrin are also used at times. These medications serve to improve mood and to allow for response to interventions. Tricyclic antidepressants are less frequently used because of their increased side effects and the potential for suicide. These medications include Elavil and Tofranil. In all cases, these medications are a start, rather than the end, of an intervention. For maximum improvement, it is critical that environmental and emotional support also be provided.

CONCLUSION

Interventions can be provided on many levels, including environmental, direct academic skills remediation, behavioral, and physiological. Each of these levels can interact with the others and result in improvement or frustration. Therefore, it is very important that home and school communicate about the child's progress, or lack thereof, on a regular basis. Although the science of these interventions is established, application of the research results continues to be an art that must be adjusted as the child develops or as new skills are required for performance.

Although there is little evidence for the applicability of the various interventions to children with TBI, they have been found to be quite successful with children with other types of disabilities. It is important to use a hypothesis-testing approach to remediation for these children, as we do not know as much about them as we know about children with learning disabilities. The most important people on the treatment team remain the special and regular education teachers. Adjustment of curricula, observations of the child's progress, and intuition provide the most appropriate interventions. A team approach that employs the strengths of various professionals can also be quite helpful. Consultation of the regular education teacher with the speech pathologist, occupational therapist, and/or physical therapist can prove invaluable. Continuing communication with the child's physician provides a bridge between the medical, rehabilitation, and school systems. Finally, the involvement of the child and parent in the program gives further support to the program as a whole and models for the child a brainstorming and problem-solving process.

The next chapter of this book offers a full case study of a young child who suffered a TBI. A case history and assessment are provided in Chapter 9. In addition, follow-up findings are presented for 2 years following the injury.

CHAPTER 9

♦♦♦

Case Illustration

♦

BACKGROUND INFORMATION

Ben was a 10-year 6-month-old male who had suffered a head injury at the age of 3 due to a major car accident in which he was a passenger in the back seat. He had hit the left side of his head against the car window and was unconscious when paramedics arrived at the scene. He was rushed to the hospital with an initial Glasgow Coma Scale (GCS) score of 4. The examination by a physician found unequal pupils, the left larger than the right, and a right parietal contusion. The diagnosis was a probable left epidural hematoma and a right hemiparesis; a CT scan was ordered. The CT report indicated a large skull fracture over the left parietal area with extensive swelling present. Surgery was performed to remove the hematoma in the left parietal region and to reconstruct the fractures involving the left parietal skull. A large, acute clot was found during the surgery, with active bleeding from a middle artery. In addition, several smaller fracture fragments were slightly depressed. A CT scan following the operation found that the hematoma had been totally removed in the left parietal lobe. Edema and contusion were also seen from the left parietal lobe to the left occipital lobe underlying the area of injury. No hemorrhage was noted, and ventricular size was normal.

A physical therapy evaluation shortly after the surgery found that Ben did not react to his right side when stimulated and showed a decreased grasp reflex on the right and no spontaneous reaching. Ben was observed to bear weight on the right, but he was unable to take steps unassisted. An occupational therapy evaluation following surgery also found right-sided difficulty, and therapy was recommended. Nursing recommendations included individual and couple counseling and parenting classes. Ben was discharged from the hospital 2 weeks after the accident.

Ben was seen in follow-up approximately 1 month after discharge. Improvement was noted, with continued mild right-sided paralysis. Results of a skull X-ray 4 months after the accident were within normal limits. At follow-up 1 year later, improvement was noted and language development was thought to be normal. Left- and right-sided skills appeared to be equal.

A developmental evaluation at age 5 indicated no areas of concern, fine and gross motor skills appeared to be within normal limits. Ben was recommended for enrollment in kindergarten that coming fall. During the summer Ben suffered a seizure, which was described as generalized. The seizure lasted approximately 10 minutes, and Ben then attempted to talk to his parents. By the time an ambulance came, Ben was seizing again and continued to do so until his arrival at the ER. He was given Valium, and the tonic–clonic activity ended, but there were persistent nystagmus, nonresponse to painful stimulation, and intermittent rhythmic arm jerking. He was given Dilantin and the Valium was repeated. The seizure activity ended after the second dose of Valium, but the nystagmus and unresponsiveness continued. He was prescribed Valium and then switched to Tegretol. A CT scan found a low-density irregular area in the white matter of the left occipital lobe, thought to be related to the previous trauma or to a congenital or intrauterine event. An EEG revealed diffuse cerebral abnormality, but no epileptogenic disturbance was noted. A repeat EEG 2 weeks later showed a disturbance of function in the left parietal occipital lobe. The neurologist suggested that these activities were potentially epileptogenic, but there were also findings suggesting a skull defect in that area. Eighteen months later Ben reported tonic–clonic movements in his right leg. This seizure was the first since his beginning Tegretol. An increase of Tegretol was recommended.

Ben was reevaluated by a neurologist at age 8 and found to show attentional difficulties, impaired fine and gross motor skills, particularly on the right, and cognitive difficulty. Memory problems were noted, and the neurologist recommended a neuropsychological evaluation at that time. No evaluation had been conducted prior to this point.

Medical History and Developmental History

Ben was the product of a full-term, uncomplicated pregnancy. His birth weight was 7 pounds 2 ounces, and a normal neonatal course was reported. Ben lives with his mother, father, and two sisters. His mother reported that Ben is very close to his father.

Educational History

Ben participated in a preschool program. School records indicate that he was verbal, and his receptive language appeared to be normal for his age.

Social skills were age-appropriate, as were his preacademic skills. Some assistance was needed for fine motor and math readiness skills. He entered kindergarten and scored in the low average range as compared with his classmates. His progress was adequate, but difficulties were noted in his attention span, which were thought to be interfering with his learning. He was diagnosed with ADHD, and Ritalin was prescribed.

In first grade, difficulty was noted in Ben's reading skills. He was referred for a multidisciplinary assessment in the winter of his first-grade year because of inconsistent general readiness skills. Psychological assessment by the school psychologist at that time indicated overall cognitive functioning in the low average range, with weaknesses in memory and information processing. Expressive language and vocabulary skills were reported to be relative strengths for Ben. Achievement testing indicated reading and math skills to be in the below average to average range. Speech and language skills were found to be within age expectations. An occupational therapy evaluation found weaknesses in sensory integration. Recommendations were for placement in a program for TBI with occupational therapy provided as well. Ben's most recent Individualized Education Plan (IEP) was reviewed in the winter of his fourth-grade year. Progress in the main academic skills has been described as limited, and attentional areas repeatedly mentioned as a main concern of his parents and teachers.

Behavioral Observations

Ben was evaluated in three sessions lasting approximately 3 hours each. He was strongly left-handed throughout the evaluation. Ben was accompanied by his parents and separated easily from them. He was appropriately groomed and of average height and weight. He was friendly and outgoing throughout the sessions. He attempted all tasks and worked his best. Ben did not take his Ritalin prior to the first testing session, but was administered 5 mg of Ritalin per the neurologist's recommendation prior to the second session. Although he was easily distracted by noises outside the room on both days, Ben could be readily redirected to the tasks at hand. He spontaneously conversed, and his language and speech were observed to be well developed for his age. Ben reported that he had great difficulty keeping his attention on his schoolwork but generally felt that school was going well. When asked why he thought he was being evaluated, he replied that it was to see what he could do and what was a problem for him. In light of Ben's good cooperation, the following results are thought to be a reliable and valid reflection of his current level of neuropsychological functioning.

TEST RESULTS AND INTERPRETATION

Tests Administered

The tests administered included the Differential Abilities Scales (DAS), Wide Range Assessment of Memory and Learning (WRAML), Wisconsin Card Sorting Test (WCST), Verbal Fluency, Trailmaking Tests A and B, Halstead–Reitan Neuropsychological Batteries, Test of Word Fluency, Test of Variables of Attention (TOVA), Grooved Pegboard, Finger Tapping, Developmental Test of Visual–Motor Integration (VMI), Judgment of Line Orientation Test (JLO), Revised Children's Manifest Anxiety Scale (RCMAS), and Children's Depression Inventory (CDI), Clinical Interview.

Cognitive Functioning

The DAS consists of core and diagnostic tests of general cognitive ability and an academic section. The cognitive subtests assess the child's ability to understand and use language, complete puzzles and block designs, and interpret visual information. The diagnostic subtests evaluate the child's short- and long-term memory and his/her speed of information processing. Average standard scores for the general cognitive index are between 85 and 115, and average T scores for the individual subtests are between 40 and 60.

	Standard score	Percentile
Verbal Cluster	84	18
Nonverbal Reasoning	83	13
Spatial	74	4
Special Nonverbal Composite	76	5
General Cognitive Ability	78	7
Core subtests	T score	Percentile
Verbal subtests		
Word Definitions	37	10
Similarities	47	38
Spatial subtests		
Recall of Designs	31	3
Pattern Construction	38	12
Nonverbal reasoning subtests		
Matrices	46	34
Sequential and Quantitative Reasoning	35	7
Diagnostic subtests		
Recall of Digits	39	14
Recall of Objects—Immediate	26	1
Recall of Objects—Delayed	28	1
Speed of Information Processing	38	12

Ben achieved a General Conceptual Ability (GCA) of 78 on the DAS, which places him in the below average range of ability and at the 7th national percentile for his age. Ben's verbal scores are generally in the average to below average range for his age, and his nonverbal reasoning and spatial skills are in the below average to significantly below average range and contributed to the below average GCA.

Ben's performance on the verbal subtests varies from below average to average. His ability to define words is below average, and his ability to reason using verbal cues is within the average range. Similarly, on the nonverbal reasoning subtests, Ben shows average skills on tasks that require him to comprehend patterns. In contrast to this performance, he shows relative weakness on tasks requiring an ability to use quantitative and sequential reasoning. Ben's spatial reasoning skills are uniformly below average, with weaknesses in visual memory and in ability to reconstruct block designs.

On the diagnostic tests Ben shows significant weaknesses in memory and below-average performance in his ability to process information quickly.

Achievement Functioning

The academic subtests of the DAS measure the child's word-reading skills, spelling, and basic number ability. Average scores fall between 85 and 115 and can be compared with the child's GCA of the DAS core subtests. Ben's scores were as follows:

	Standard score	Percentile
Basic Number Skills	70	2
Spelling	68	2
Word Reading	64	1

Ben shows below average performance on tasks measuring his ability to perform arithmetical calculation and to spell words. His word-reading skills are significantly below average for his age and his ability level. These findings are consistent with school records and previous testing.

Memory Functioning

The WRAML is a measure that assesses the child's ability to recall information both verbally and visually presented. The WRAML provides a screening form that evaluates the child's ability to notice changes in a picture, recall a visual design after a short interval, learn a list of unrelated words over several trials, and recall a story that is read to the child. Average standard scores are between 85 and 115, and average scaled scores are between 7 and 13. Ben's scores were as follows:

	Standard score	Percentile
Memory Screening Index	86	18

	Scaled score
Picture Memory	11
Design Memory	6
Verbal Learning	7
Story Memory	8
Sentence Memory	8
Visual Learning	5

Ben shows overall memory skills in the low average range for his age. His ability to remember visual information presented in a context (picture memory) is significantly stronger than his ability to recall nonmeaningful designs or to remember information presented spatially. Ben's ability to remember a story and sentences is within the average range for his age. His memory for a list of unrelated words is in the low-average range. Ben shows the ability to retain information learned, as measured by the delayed recall subtests for the Story Memory, Verbal Learning, and Visual Learning subtests.

Executive Functioning

The WCST is a measure of executive functioning, including the ability to form concepts, generate an organizational strategy, and use examiner feedback to shift strategy to the changing demands of the task. Average standard scores range from 85 to 115. Ben's performance is summarized in the following table:

	Standard score	Percentile
Total Number of Errors	102	55
Perseverative Errors	116	86
Nonperseverative Errors	90	25
Number of Categories Achieved	6	Above average
Trials to Complete First Category	0	Above average
Failure to Maintain Set	0	Above average

Ben shows average to above average scores on the WCST. He was able to understand the problem, figure out alternative solutions, and maintain the solution he had found even when distracting stimuli were presented.

The Test of Word Fluency (FAS) was also administered. This task requires the child to name as many words as possible beginning with a specified letter within a 1-minute time span. The child first names words beginning with *F*, then *A*, then *S*. Ben showed significant difficulty on this task, and his z score was −1.6 (between −1.00 and +1.00 is average). He had difficulty recalling words beginning with *A* and was unable to retrieve additional words from his memory.

The Category test of the Halstead–Reitan was also administered. Ben scored in the above average range for his age, getting 51 correct. He showed good problem-solving ability on this test. Trailmaking, a measure of mental flexibility, was found to be in the average range for Ben's age.

Attentional Functioning

The TOVA is a computerized measure of visual sustained attention and provides indices of sustained attention, impulsivity, response time, and variability of response. Average standard scores are between 85 and 115. The TOVA was administered with Ben off Ritalin but on Tegretol, and on 5 mg of Ritalin. His scores were as follows:

	Off Ritalin	On 5 mg Ritalin
Omission (Inattention)	85	76[a]
Commission (Impulsivity)	86	102
Response Time	87	84
Variability	55[a]	70

[a]Outside average limits.

Ben showed low average performance on all measures except variability while off Ritalin. On 5 mg of Ritalin he showed good improvement in impulsivity and variability, although the variability score continued to be outside normal limits. On Ritalin, Ben showed improved ability to control his responses, as noted by the decrease in multiple button presses. His inattention score declined slightly, most predominantly due to difficulty in the second half of the test when stimuli are presented more quickly. He appeared motivated to complete the task. It may well be that the 5 mg of Ritalin, which is less than his usual dose, does not provide sufficient medication to improve his attention even with good effort.

A clinical interview with Ben's parents indicated that he meets DSM-IV criteria for attention-deficit/hyperactivity disorder, combined type. His parents reported a number of symptoms: problems in maintaining attention, following through on instructions, organization; not listening to what is being said to him, losing things necessary to complete a task, being forgetful; being overactive; and impulse control. His teacher also reported that Ben shows difficulty with attention, restlessness, and difficulty in finishing his work. Both parents are concerned about Ben's taking medication, but his mother stated that if medication was warranted, they would support his taking it.

Motor Functioning

The Grooved Pegboard is a motor task that requires the child to place pegs into keys arranged on a board. The test provides measures of motor quickness as well as errors. Scores are converted to z scores, and average performance is between –1.0 and +1.0. Higher positive scores are not desirable. Ben used his left hand as his preferred hand on this task. His scores were as follows:

Dominant Hand Time	+0.78	Average
Dominant Hand Errors	0	
Nondominant Hand Time	+0.96	Low Average
Nondominant Hand Errors	0	Average

Ben scored in the average range for his age on this task. He experienced significantly more difficulty with his right hand and had difficulty picking up the pegs. He was diligent in working on this task, and his motivation certainly assisted his performance.

The Finger Tapping test is a motor task that requires the child to tap on a metal key as quickly as possible for 10 seconds without removing his hand from the board to which the key is attached. A mean of three trials is obtained. Scores are converted to z scores, and average performance is between –1.0 and +1.0. Scores in the high positive range are not desirable. Ben used his left hand as his preferred hand on this task. His scores were as follows:

Dominant Hand	+0.11	Average
Nondominant Hand	Unable to complete	

Ben showed average performance on this task with his left hand. He experienced significant difficulty with his right hand and was unable to keep his palm on the board and to avoid moving his other fingers while doing the task. Therefore, this portion of the task was not completed in light of the standardization requirements for the test.

The Grip Strength test also indicated significant difficulties with the right hand. Ben achieved the following scores:

Dominant Hand	24.5 kilograms	Average
Nondominant Hand	2.5 kilograms	Significantly below average

The VMI is a measure of the child's ability to copy increasingly more complex figures. Ben achieved a score in the below average range and at the 13th national percentile for his age. He had difficulty with orientation of the designs.

The JLO asks the child to match two lines to an array of lines. This task requires visual perceptual skills and visual discrimination. Scores are converted to z scores, and average scores are between +1.0 and −1.0. High negative scores indicate poorer performance. Ben achieved a score of −1.86, which is significantly below average for his age. These scores are consistent with Ben's performance on the DAS spatial abilities subtests.

The Tactual Performance Test (TPT) of the Halstead–Reitan indicated weakness with his right hand and average performance with his left hand. When both hands were used together, Ben performed in the average range. Memory skills were found to be within normal ranges for his age, and memory for spatial location significantly below average.

These areas of weakness are consistent with difficulty in the parietal lobe. The parietal lobe is believed to be responsible for spatial reasoning as well as visual–motor functioning. Particular difficulty was noted in motor overflow and fine motor dexterity with Ben's right hand.

Sensory–Perceptual Functioning

Ben showed age-appropriate skills in his ability to localize touch to his face and hands bilaterally. He had difficulty in localizing his fingers, particularly on his right hand. His errors on this test were consistent and on all fingers except his thumb. These difficulties were also noted in the fingertip writing task for the right hand, with 16 errors out of 20 presentations. These findings are consistent with Ben's difficulty in sensory interpretation with his right hand. Although attention problems can interfere with performance on this task, Ben's difficulty appeared to be more related to interpreting sensory information with his right hand. His performance with his left hand yielded no errors.

Emotional Functioning

Ben's emotional functioning was screened to determine his adjustment. He scored in the average range on the CDI. He reported no significant areas of difficulty on this measure. Because of Ben's reading problems, the test was read to him.

The RCMAS is a self-report measure to evaluate a child's feelings about him/herself. Ben scored in the average range on all measures of the RCMAS, indicating no significant areas of concern.

The Behavior Assessment System for Children (BASC) was also administered to his parents. The BASC is an integrated system designed to facilitate the differential diagnosis and classification of a variety of emotional and behavioral disorders of children and to aid in the design of treatment plans. Ben's mother's responses on this measure were consistent with her report of his behavior on interview and with school reports. T scores are reported in the following table, with an average of 50 and the average range between 40 and 60. Scores between 60 and 70 on the BASC are considered to indicate an "at risk" condition for the development of further problems. Percentile ranks are also reported.

Domain	T score	Percentile
Hyperactivity	76[a]	99
Aggression	69[b]	95
Conduct Problems	50	50
Externalizing Problems	69[a]	85
Anxiety	57	77
Depression	57	77
Somatization	53	68
Internalizing Problems	56	75
Atypicality	56	75
Withdrawal	58	77
Attention Problems	73[b]	98
Behavioral Symptoms Index	66[a]	92
Higher scores are desirable on the following scales:		
Adaptability	45	35
Social Skills	50	50
Leadership	45	35
Adaptive Skills Composite	46	43

[a]Clinically significant; [b]at-risk behaviors.

Ben's teacher also completed the BASC. She indicated concerns very similar to those of Ben's mother. Difficulties in attention and hyperactivity were noted. Areas of concern were that Ben had difficulty staying on task, frequently forgot directions, experienced problems completing seatwork and homework, and frequently interrupted peers and adults.

Domain	T score	Percentile
Hyperactivity	69[a]	95
Aggression	68[a]	93
Conduct Problems	51	71
Externalizing Problems	64[a]	90
Anxiety	55	76
Depression	55	76
Somatization	55	77
Internalizing Problems	55	76
Attention Problems	73[b]	99
Learning Problems	67[a]	93
School Problems	70[b]	96
Atypicality	58	80
Withdrawal	55	76
Behavioral Symptoms Index	69[a]	94

For the following scales, higher scores are desirable:

Adaptability	40	14
Social Skills	41	18
Leadership	41	18
Study Skills	35[a]	8
Adaptive Skills	40	14

[a]At-risk behaviors; [b]clinically significant.

Ben also completed the BASC—Self-Report. He denied any areas of concern, and many of his scores are lower than would be expected of a child his age. As compared with his profile, Ben's interpersonal relationships were significantly lower than his other scores, indicating some concern on his part about his relationships with his peers. Ben's scores are as follows:

Domain	Standard score	Percentile
Attitude to School	46	43
Attitude to Teachers	49	56
School Maladjustment	47	47
Atypicality	43	29
Locus of Control	55	67
Social Stress	54	66
Anxiety	55	66
Depression	53	70
Sense of Inadequacy	59	82
Clinical Maladjustment	52	60
Emotional Symptoms Index	55	72

For the following scales, higher scores are desirable:

Relations with Parents	57	76
Interpersonal Relations	40	15
Self-Esteem	57	73
Self-Reliance	54	58
Personal Adjustment	53	48

IMPRESSIONS AND RECOMMENDATIONS

Ben is a 10-year 6-month-old white male who experienced a severe head injury at age 3 years in a motor vehicle accident. Medical records indicate a loss of consciousness as well as significant signs of head trauma. Neurosurgery was necessary to evacuate a hematoma, and right-sided paresis resulted after the injury. Ben received physical and occupational therapy following the accident, and his family received nursing support. Ben experienced a seizure at age 6 and was placed on Tegretol.

Evaluations in school indicated significant difficulties in learning and attention, and Ben was diagnosed with ADHD in first grade and put on Ritalin. He was evaluated by his school district, and a multidisciplinary team found him to have exceptional educational needs and recommended placement in a program for children with TBI. He has received services in reading, math, written language, and occupational therapy since first grade.

Ben's current evaluation indicates strengths in the areas of abstract verbal and visual reasoning, with significant weakness in sequential and quantitative reasoning, in spatial and design memory, and in short-term memory for nonmeaningful verbal information. Particular difficulty was found in his ability to learn by using visual cues and relative strength in remembering verbal information when presented in context. Ben's fine motor coordination and control were found to be mildly to moderately affected, particularly with his right hand. His ability to solve novel problems and to be cognitively flexible is well within the average range for his age. Ben's academic skills show significant weaknesses in reading and spelling and below average performance on mathematics tasks. No emotional difficulties were identified. Ben continues to qualify for a diagnosis of ADHD, combined type.

Ben's pattern of weaknesses is consistent with damage to the left parieto-occipital association areas. Spatial and visual integration abilities are generally attributed to this region of the brain. His memory for nonmeaningful information, both visually and orally presented, is poor and negatively affects his ability to learn new facts if they are not presented within a framework (i.e., single-word reading). In addition, Ben shows at least average ability on measures of reasoning, indicating that he would have had at least average overall ability without the head trauma and may not have had the learning disabilities he now has.

His development up to the point of the accident was reported to be normal, and there is no familial history of learning disabilities or ADHD. The presence of ADHD may or may not be due to the accident, but it likely exacerbates his difficulties in learning and in memory. Because of his young age, it was not possible to accurately determine whether ADHD was present before the accident, and parent reports indicate no concern in that area. However, the motor findings do implicate the left frontal region and may suggest disruption in this region and in subcortically related areas. It is possible that Ben's ADHD was triggered by the accident, given the difficulty with psychomotor speed/processing speed and attentional deficits.

In light of the preceding findings, the following recommendations are offered:

1. It is recommended that Ben's parents consider continuing his current medication regimen. He shows a response to the medication, according to his parents report, and without adequate medication Ben is highly distractible and experiences considerable difficulty in staying on task.

2. It is further recommended that Ben be neuropsychologically evaluated yearly in order to document his progress, adjust recommendations and treatment interventions, and monitor any difficulties that may arise as he gets older.

3. Ben's teachers and the school system are to be commended for providing a good special education program for him. It is suggested that his program continue and services be provided as needed for Ben's success. His reading program should emphasize reading for content rather than relying on rote memory of words. It will be important to provide Ben with additional tutoring in reading to improve his skills. His reading ability appears to be improved with the use of phonics, and a phonics-based program appears most appropriate. In addition, his textbooks in science and social studies should be tape-recorded so that he can listen to the content without the added burden of having to decode the words.

4. Memory strategies are crucial for Ben's success, and he needs support in developing this type of compensation. It is important that these strategies be directly taught. The ability to remember items is frequently enhanced by teaching the child to associate new learning with something he already knows. Rote memorization will be quite difficult for Ben. Thus, for mathematics facts, sight word vocabulary, and the like, it will be most helpful to provide visual cues as well as practice until these skills become automatized. In addition, there are several good computer programs that provide drill without being boring. Study skills that use memory may also be helpful. For example, the PQRST strategy guides study through a mnemonic:

Previewing the order of the text or chapter,
Questioning the main point addressed by the material,
Reading the chapter carefully,
Stating the premise of what has been read, and
Testing for understanding.

External aids are methods used to extend or supplement internal storage mechanisms. Examples include lists, diaries, notebooks, computers, portable timers, and electronic calculators.

5. Ben needs to improve his attentional skills. The following suggestions are offered to assist teachers and parents with his program.

Environmental considerations
a. Assign Ben priority seating.
b. Ensure that there are few distractions.
c. Seat Ben away from peers with similar problems.
d. Allow Ben to go to a distraction-free area to complete work requiring additional attention.

Lesson and worksheets

a. Provide Ben with advance organizers for lessons; provide key vocabulary prior to the lessons for review at home or with his special education teacher.

b. Worksheets should be reduced to the amount of information that is most important for Ben to learn. If necessary, worksheets should be cut up to provide fewer distractions.

c. Tests should be administered orally and Ben should be provided with additional time to think of his answers.

d. Writing is difficult for Ben, so provision of alternatives may be necessary. Classes in keyboarding are particularly important for Ben and may offer the additional support he needs.

e. Ben may respond better to tasks that require cooperative, rather than competitive, learning skills. Pairing him with a group of students of varying abilities will be most helpful.

f. The use of colored chalk may assist Ben in paying attention to the most important parts of a lesson.

g. Worksheets should use larger type, and the contrast should be good.

h. Key direction words, vocabulary, and important concepts should be highlighted for Ben.

6. Ben will also need some assistance with his writing skills. He should be evaluated for assistive technology. It would be quite helpful for him to enroll in keyboarding classes and to be given an outline of the class material.

Reevaluation

For the year following his evaluation at age 10 years 6 months, Ben continued in his special education program, with additional support provided in writing and sensory–motor skills. The IEP that was developed following this evaluation included recommendations for additional reading support and assistance in mathematics. His regular education teacher began using graph paper to assist Ben in aligning columns for his mathematics problems. Ben also enrolled in a keyboarding class to assist with his writing. His school district provided him with a notebook computer on which to take notes during class.

Ben was reevaluated at age 12 to determine his progress. Assessment at that time indicated a full scale IQ of 87 on the WISC-III (verbal IQ 90; performance IQ 83). Subtests indicated average vocabulary and reasoning skills with significant weaknesses in perceptual organization, short-term memory, and arithmetic reasoning. Achievement testing continued to show weaknesses in reading and spelling, with improvement in mathematics cal-culation and reasoning. His reading recognition skills were measured at a standard score of 67 on the Wide Range Achievement Test-3 (WRAT-3) and spelling at 71. Arithmetic was at 85.

The WRAML was readministered and showed average performance in verbal and visual skills (96 and 107, respectively), with below average skills again noted on the learning index (80). Delayed memory and verbal recall were found to be in the average range, with sound symbols being signifi-cantly below average for his age. Story recognition skills were found to be in the average range. At this time the California Verbal Learning Test—Children's Version (CVLT-C) was also administered with Ben on medica-tion, and the following results were found:

	Raw score	Standard score
List A, Trial 1	4	−1.0
List A, Trial 5	8	−1.5
Trials 1 to 5	36	−1.0
List B, Free Recall	3	−1.5
List A, Short Delay Free Recall	8	−0.5
List A, Short Delay Cued Recall	9	−0.5
List A, Long Delay Free Recall	9	−0.5
List A, Long Delay Cued Recall	9	−0.5
Correct Recognition Hits	12	−0.5
Discriminability	91.11%	0.0
Learning Slope	1.3	0.0

Ben's performance on the CVLT-C indicated that he has poor initial ability to encode information in working memory. He was below average in his ability to acquire verbal material through repetition. Thus, he repeated four words after initial exposure, but acquired only four further words af-ter four repetitions. He also had some difficulty in recall after a short delay. These difficulties may be based in problems with retrieval processes, as Ben was able to correctly recognize words that were on the list and successfully discriminated them from distractor words that were not on the list. This good discriminability suggests that although Ben was encoding the list ini-tially, the difficulty he experienced was in successfully retrieving and ex-pressing what had been encoded. Moreover, Ben did not use particularly ef-ficient strategies for retrieval, relying on the serial positioning of the words on the list (and recalling those at the end of the list most often) rather than clustering them into semantically related categories.

The findings derived from the memory measures have important impli-cations for Ben's school performance. First, Ben displays below average ability to learn new information through repeated exposure without the aid of concrete cues. Therefore, in the classroom he will most likely learn material at a much slower rate than other children. He did not spontaneously generate efficient strategies for encoding and may have to be taught more effective means of remembering new material. It also appears that new learning may be taking place but that Ben is having difficulty with retrieval. Thus, he should be provided with a system of cueing himself to help him remember information he has just learned. In addition, new learning should be rehearsed often to help render retrieval somewhat easier.

A modified Halstead–Reitan Battery was readministered to evaluate Ben's motor skills and to reevaluate his perceptual abilities. Ben's performance on the TPT indicated average performance bilaterally, with average skills in memory for designs and low average skills in memory for spatial location. The sensory–perceptual/motor examination found performance to be within normal limits for Ben's age. No significant visual, tactile, auditory, or sensory difficulties were found. Finger tapping and grip strength remained below average for Ben's right hand, particularly in comparison to age norms and to his performance with his left hand.

The Bender–Gestalt was also administered, and Ben's drawings were basically within normal limits. Some difficulty was found in impulsive responding.

Taken together, these findings continue to implicate the left hemisphere, particularly in the frontal regions, with possible interconnections to subcortical regions such as the basal ganglia. Continued difficulty with sound–symbol relationships was found, and skills in this province are generally related to difficulty in the association areas of the parietal, occipital, and temporal regions—regions affected by Ben's accident. Given his age of 12, it is likely that he will not improve dramatically in his basic reading skills, particularly in light of the amount of extra reading support he has received since first grade. Therefore, it was recommended that reading skills be supported through books on tape, allowing Ben to give oral answers to tests, and to tape-record any essay questions. It was also strongly suggested that support be provided through peer note taking in his classes and that resource room support be continued.

There has been improvement in his motor skills, and Ben has become adept in his use of the computer notebook. Written work was reduced to demonstrating mastery of concepts. Support for memory skills was also provided, with an organizer utilized to recall classwork assignments and appointments. Direct work in helping Ben organize information continued to assist him in his transition to middle school. It was also recommended that Ben participate in the program that allowed for block scheduling, whereby he would have fewer class transitions each day. Classes were scheduled on alternative days and for longer periods of time.

Ben, his parents, and his teacher continued to report improvement when Ben was administered Ritalin. The BASC completed by his special education and regular education science teachers indicated average performance when he was on medication. Ben had not experienced any seizures in the past three years, and his neurologist was beginning the process of weaning him off Tegretol. In regard to this plan, a meeting was called with Ben's major regular education teachers, his special education teacher, Ben, and his parents, with input from his pediatrician as to the effects of this process on Ben's learning skills. A contingency plan was developed for the unlikely possibility of a seizure occurring during the weaning process.

Ben's physical and occupational therapists had dismissed him from direct services but continued to serve as consultants on an as-needed basis. Ben's parents reported that their family therapy had been successfully terminated the previous year. Ben had formed friendships in his classes and had become active in the soccer program despite continued weakness on his right side. It was recommended that Ben's program be reevaluated in his freshman year in high school to determine additional needs that may have arisen, and to develop an individualized transition plan at age 16.

CHAPTER 10

◆◆◆

Parting Thoughts

◆

This book has attempted to provide a background in traumatic brain injury (TBI) in the pediatric population. As such, it has reviewed the basic neuroanatomy needed to understand neurological and neuroradiological reports, described frequently used neuropsychological measures, made suggestions for testing that can be completed by a psychologist without extensive neuropsychological training, and presented classroom and family interventions that are used in the field. In reviewing the body of work on TBI, it was amazing to discover how few studies are reported on the efficacy of interventions in frequent use. Although there are several good books describing educational interventions (e.g., Savage & Wolcott, 1988), the empirical evidence backing these prescriptive writings is missing. Good teachers certainly are readily able to adjust materials for children experiencing learning difficulties. However, it is reassuring for teachers to know that what they are doing has some empirical foundation. This area of research is important and desperately requires more investigation.

Before anyone can begin to prescribe treatment, educational or medical, it is generally helpful to carefully determine and understand the parameters of a disorder and the impact it may have on everyday life. There is sufficient disagreement about the sequelae of mild head injury to make one stop and think about what children and adolescents with TBI may be experiencing. Over the years, I have evaluated several children with mild head injury and have generally found few frank neuropsychological deficits. However, the childrens' parents frequently described behavioral difficulties and emotional lability that were not present prior to the injury, suggesting that some problems may be due to the injury, which we are unable to measure because of their subtlety. Emerging research indicates that it is very important to evaluate children's premorbid behavioral functioning, as those with problematic behaviors prior to injury appear to continue with behavioral difficulty after the accident. However, after the accident some may attribute behavioral problems to that the incident rather than realizing that they were present prior to the injury. Although some behaviors may have been present prior to the injury, it is important not to assume that the behavioral difficulties seen after the accident are of the same magnitude or intensity.

In this situation a very good interview can assist in delving into the behaviors and determining the effect of a child's premorbid status on his/her postinjury functioning. It is not only useful in assisting school and community agencies to help the child but also in helping the family to understand the child's behaviors. Too often parents I worked with thought that the behaviors were immutable, and therefore interventions were believed to be ineffective. However, when a cognitive–behavioral program or a similarly structured therapy has been established, improvement has been seen. It is important to empower not only the family, but also the child, and to encourage them in believing that change can occur. Children with ADHD have been found to have a higher than expected incidence of head injury. It is likely that the disorder may be more disruptive following such an injury, partially because of the stress felt by the family. Complicating matters even further, many families that have children with ADHD also have parents with ADHD. I remember one father coming up to me after a workshop I conducted on TBI and saying, "Peg, the recommendations for organization and attention were quite helpful—but many of you forget that many of us parents have ADHD too." It is important to remember this father's statement when working with families and to accommodate the difficulties that may be present within the family structure as well as in the child.

MILD HEAD INJURY

Our knowledge of the effects of mild and moderate head injury is not in the depth we might wish. Levin and colleagues are seeking to evaluate children with TBI using a multimethod, multi-informant system. Such a system takes into account the behaviors seen prior to the accident and those seen as a result of the injury.

Pennington (1991) provides a model that discusses the primary, cor related, and artifactual symptoms associated with disorders such as ADHD and learning disabilities. This model may be helpful in understanding severe head injury as well. It is possible that the primary symptoms may include memory, attention, and motor difficulties, with correlated deficits including behavioral difficulties, learning problems, and social deficits.

Artifactual symptoms may include delinquency, substance abuse, and family discord. The use of this model for mild head injury may also assist us in understanding that symptoms are related and in determining which of them co-occur because of other problems. For example, children with mild head injury may be found to initially show some emotional distress and may also appear disinhibited. Attentional and memory problems are also reported in the literature. If a child is unable to pay attention, he/she will be unable to recall what was learned. This difficulty is frequently seen in TBI. It would be helpful to establish which of these symptoms are primary and which are correlated in the same manner as in children with severe head injuries.

FAMILY

The strengths of the family to help the child reintegrate into his/her everyday living situation are a resource that should be recognized and utilized. However, it is also important to assess how much one can ask of a family. Too many clinicians appear to use the shotgun approach—that is, they include every possible recommendation, from individual therapy to family therapy to psychopharmocology to academic remediation. I have witnessed families attempting to use all of these resources and being run ragged. This state of affairs can also happen in the school setting with programs set up by well-meaning educators. One child who was a client of mine was in so many therapies that he was in his classroom for only 1 hour a day, which left little time for learning or socializing. Although these therapies are valuable and important, it is also important not to overwhelm the child and the family with too many things at one time. It is reasonable to determine the priority of needs and to reach an agreement with the family about what should be done now and what can wait.

In addition, research indicates that families often do not reach out for help when they are experiencing the greatest emotional distress. It is important to be cognizant of this tendency, particularly for those of us who work in schools. It is also important to recognize that families may distrust professionals and may have had some experiences during the child's recovery that make them pull away from such help. School–home partnerships are particularly important and require nurturing throughout the evaluation and remediation process. A consultation process that recognizes the value of the parents' input can be helpful in establishing lines of communication. In the medical model the expert tells the parent what to do. Although this system may work within a hospital or other medical setting, it does not readily translate to the school situation and should be avoided wherever possible.

THERAPY ISSUES

Sometimes professionals are so dedicated to assisting the child that they may lose sight of what the child can manage. Earlier I mentioned a child who was in so many therapies that there was little time for socialization or even learning in the regular classroom. It is very difficult to balance the various requirements of children's educational needs with their very real need to be "normal." In designing a program, however, it is important that the professionals pay attention to balance. It may be difficult for an occupational therapist or speech therapist to report that right now other therapies should take precedence and his/her therapy may have to wait. Thus, it may be appropriate for various therapies to be scheduled prior to or after the school day. Yet balance should not be at the convenience of the school system and should certainly not be used to excuse the lack of service to the child. What I am suggesting is that all professionals consider the schedule the child is expected to follow and determine whether it is *realistic*.

TRAINING ISSUES

Another area that needs development is training. For many school psychologists and child clinical psychologists one course in physiological psychology is required. Courses in neuropsychology, biological bases of behavior, or neuroanatomy are usually attended only by students who have a specific interest in the area. Given the number of children with TBI and other childhood neurological disorders (tumors, leukemia, cancer, spina bifida, etc.) that require an understanding of neuropsychology, it appears important for students to be provided with at least an overview of this area. At the very least, one course in neuropsychology would be important in the preparation of these professionals. Programs that provide courses in neuroanatomy, neuropsychology, and psychopharmocology prepare students to better understand the complex cases that are now seen in schools and clinics. Children with serious neurological disorders did not survive in the near past, but now, even with some changes in neuropsychological functioning, live normal life spans. It is also important that students who are interested in neuropsychology be provided an opportunity to take courses in child and adult neuropsychology. As mentioned earlier, students may be provided only one course, and if it is adult neuropsychology, many assume that they can apply the principles of adult neuropsychology to children. This assumption ignores the differences between children and adults and may lead to the inappropriate application of skills developed for adults to children and young adolescents.

Thus, it is important for the school professional, as well as the child clinical psychologist, to understand the complex nature of head injury. School psychologists are in a unique position to provide services for children with TBI. New fields, such as school pediatric psychology, also serve as bridges between the medical and educational worlds. It is an exciting time to work as a school psychologist, child clinical psychologist, or pediatric neuropsychologist as our knowledge is increasing and we understand the brain in so much greater detail.

Glossary

♦

Amygdala: Structure within the limbic system that is involved in the modulation of strong emotions, including rage and fear.

Axons: Structures that carry messages away from the cell body and toward another cell body.

Basal Ganglia: Connect the cortex with midbrain structures. Implicated in motor and emotional responses.

Brainstem: Most posterior structure. Connects the brain and spinal cord. Region where most cranial nerves are located, as well as structures involved in basic life functions.

Cell Body: The life center of the neuron. Contains the basic genetic material as well as the nucleus and energy-producing structures.

Central Nervous System (CNS): Comprised of the brain and the spinal cord.

Central Sulcus: Separates the frontal lobe from the parietal lobe.

Cerebellum: Receives information about the position of limbs in space, provides balance, and allows skilled movements. Located in the posterior region of the brain above the brainstem.

Cerebrospinal Fluid (CSF): A colorless solution of sodium chloride and other salts that cushions the brain. Produced in the ventricles.

Computed Tomography (CT) Scans: Visualization of brain anatomy by means of a narrow X-ray beam.

Coup: The original area of impact of a head injury.

Contrecoup: The area opposite the head injury impact.

Corpus Callosum: The large bundle of fibers that connects the two brain hemispheres.

Dendrite: Branch of a cell body that receives impulses from other neurons.

Deoxyribonucleic acid (DNA): The genetic blueprint of a cell.

Diencephalon: Responsible for the integration of sensory experiences and relaying the resulting response.

Dura Mater: The outer covering of the central nervous system.

fMRI: Functional magnetic resonance imaging. An emerging clinical technique that allows for the mapping of cerebral blood flow, as well as changes in this flow and oxygenation.

Glasgow Coma Scale (GCS): A scale used to ascertain the level of head injury.

Gray Matter: The nuclei of the neurons.

Gyri: Ridges within the cerebrum.

Hematoma: A bruise. Can be either on the brain or in the brain.

Hippocampus: Structure located in the temporal lobe that is responsible for the laying down of new memories.

Hypothalamus: Structure responsible for modulation and control of emotions, sexual functions, eating, temperature, and thirst.

Internal Capsule: A connection between the frontal lobes and subcortical structures.

Lateral (Sylvian) Fissure: Separates the frontal lobe from the temporal lobe.

Lateralization: The extent to which each hemisphere is specialized for certain types of tasks.

Limbic System: Series of structures that serve as a relay for cognitive and emotional input.

Magnetic Resonance Imaging (MRI): A technique that allows for the viewing of internal brain structures without the use of X-rays.

Medulla Oblongata: Located in the brainstem. Contains sensory and motor nuclei as well as several of the cranial nerves.

Meninges: Lining of the brain and spinal cord. Serve to protect the central nervous system from damage.

Mild Head Injury: Head injury that results in loss of consciousness or posttraumatic amnesia of less than 1 hour and a Glasgow Coma Scale score of 13 to 15.

Mitochondria: Responsible for the energy production for the cell.

Moderate Head Injury: Head injury that results in loss of consciousness or posttraumatic amnesia lasting from 1 to 24 hours and a Glasgow Coma Scale score of 9 to 12.

Myelin: A fatty substance that covers the long axons and allows for the rapid transmission of nerve impulses.

Neuroglia: Tissue that provides structural support and insulation of the synapses between cells.

Neuron: The conductor of nerve impulses. Made up of axons, cell bodies, dendrites, and axon terminals.

Nucleus: Includes the chromosomes and nucleolus.

Nucleolus: Manufactures structures involved in protein synthesis.

Orbitofrontal Regions: The region of the frontal lobes generally in the eye sockets or orbits.

Peripheral Nervous System (PNS): Connects the central nervous system to the rest of the body through spinal, cranial, and peripheral nerves.

Pia Mater: The innermost of the meninges of the spinal cord and brain.

Pituitary Gland: Structure that releases hormones regulating bodily functions.

Pons: Located between the medulla and midbrain. A bridge between the right and left hemispheres. Major sensory and motor pathways are located here.

Posttraumatic Amnesia: The time required for a child to understand time and spatial orientation and to remember prior events following traumatic brain injury.

Primary Effects: Injury due to the accident itself.

Reticular Activating System: Structure located in the brainstem responsible for control of blood pressure, blood volume, heart rate, and consciousness.

Ribonucleic Acid (RNA): Responsible for protein synthesis. Transmits instructions about metabolism.

Secondary Effects: Injury due to swelling and contusions suffered as a result of the initial injury.

Severe Head Injury: Head injury that results in a loss of consciousness or posttraumatic amnesia for more than 24 hours with a Glasgow Coma Scale of 3 to 8.

Shearing: Damage as a result of stretching and distortion of the axons when a head injury occurs.

Subarachnoid Space: Located between the pia and the dura mater. Filled with cerebrospinal fluid.

Sulci: Valleys on the cortex.

Synapse: The space between neurons that allows impulses to travel from one neuron to another.

Temporal Poles: The most anterior section of the temporal lobe. At great risk of injury, as they lie next to the bony skull and upon impact are generally pushed into the skull.

Thalamus: Brain structure responsible for relaying visual, auditory, motor, and sensory information to the cerebrum.

Traumatic Brain Injury: Occurs when the brain impacts another object. May involve loss of consciousness.

Ventricles: Large cavities in the brain that produce cerebrospinal fluid.

White Matter: The myelinated axons of neurons. Located in the center of the brain and surrounded by gray matter.

APPENDIX

♦♦♦

Test Resources

♦

California Verbal Learning Test—Children's Revision (1994). Published by Psychological Corporation (1-800-872-1726 or on the Internet at www.psychcorp.com).

NEPSY: A Developmental Neuropsychological Assessment (1998). Published by Psychological Corporation.

D2 Test of Attention (1998). Published by Hogrefe & Huber Publishers; available also through Psychological Assessment Resources (1-800-331-TEST or on the Internet at www.parinc.com).

Wisconsin Card Sorting Test (1993). Published by Psychological Assessment Resources and many others.

Test of Memory and Learning (1995). Published by Pro-Ed (1-800-897-3202 or on the Internet at www.proedinc.com).

Children's Memory Scale (1996). Published by Psychological Corporation.

Stroop Color Word Test (1994). Published by Stoelting Company (630-860-9700 or on the Internet at www.stoeltingco.com).

Purdue Pegboard. Published by Psychological Corporation.

WISC-III PI (1999). Published by Psychological Corporation.

References

♦

Abreau, F., Templer, D. L., Schuyler, B. A., & Hutchinson, H. T. (1990). Neuropsy-chological assessment of soccer players. *Neuropsychology, 4,* 175–181.

Achenbach, T. M. (1991). *Manual for the Child Behavior Checklist.* Burlington: Department of Psychiatry, University of Vermont.

Aldenkamp, A. P. (1995). Cognitive side-effects of antiepileptic drugs. In A. P. Aldenkamp, F. E. Dreifuss, W. O. Reiner, & T. P. B. M. Suurmeijer (Eds.), *Epilepsy in children and adolescents* (pp. 161–181). Boca Raton, FL: CRC Press.

Allen, K., Linn, R. T., Gutierrez, H., & Willer, B. S. (1994). Family burdern following traumatic brain injury. *Rehabilitation Psychology, 39,* 30–48.

Alves, W. M., & Jane, J. A. (1985). Mild brain injury: Damage and outcome. In D. Becker & J. T. Povlishock (Eds.), *Central nervous system trauma: Status report* (pp. 255–271). Bethesda, MD: National Institutes of Health.

Aram, D. M., & Eisele, J. A. (1994). Intellectual stability in children with unilateral lesions. *Neuropsychologia, 32,* 85–96.

Asarnow, R. F., Satz, P., Light, R., Lewis, R., & Neumann, E. (1991). Behavior problems and adaptive functioning in children with mild and severe closed head injury. *Journal of Pediatric Psychology, 16,* 543–555.

Asarnow, R. F., Satz, P., Light, R., Zaucha, K., Lewis, R., & McCleary, C. (1995). The UCLA study of mild closed head injury in children and adolescents. In S. Broman & M. E. Michel (Eds.), *Traumatic head injury in children and adolescents* (pp. 117–146). New York: Oxford University Press.

Ashwal, S., & Schneider, S. (1994). Neurologic complications of vasculitis disorders of childhood. In K. F. Swaiman (Ed.), *Pediatric neurology* (2nd ed., pp. 780–801). St. Louis, MO: Mosby.

Bakker, D. J. (1972). *Temporal order in disturbed reading.* Rotterdam: Rotterdam University Press.

Banich, M. T., Levine, S. C., Kim, H., & Huttenlocher, P. (1990). The effects of developmental factors on IQ in hemiplegic children. *Neuropsychologia, 28,* 35–47.

Barker, L. H., Bigler, E. D., Johnson, S. C., Anderson, C. V., Russo, A. A., Boineau,

B., & Butler, D. D. (1999). Polysubstance abuse and traumatic brain injury: Quantitative magnetic resonance imaging and neuropsychological outcome in older adolescents and young adults. *Journal of the International Neuropsychological Society, 5,* 593–608.

Barkley, R. A. (1998). *Attention-deficit/hyperactivity disorder: A handbook for diagnosis and treatment* (2nd ed.). New York: Guilford Press.

Barkley, R. A. (2000). *Taking charge of ADHD: The complete, authoritative guide for parents* (Rev. ed.). New York: Guilford Press.

Barth, J. T., & Macciocchi, S. N. (1985). The Halstead–Reitan Neuropsychological Test Battery. In C. Newmark (Ed.), *Major psychological assessment techniques* (pp. 381–414). Boston: Allyn & Bacon.

Baxter, R., Cohen, S. B., & Ylvisaker, M. (1985). Comprehensive cognitive assessment. In M. Ylvisaker (Ed.), *Head injury rehabilitation: Children and adolescents* (pp. 247–274). San Diego, CA: College-Hill Press.

Beaumont, J. G. (1983). *Introduction to neuropsychology.* New York: Guilford Press.

Beery, K. E. (1990). *Revised administration, scoring, and teaching manual for the Developmental Test of Visual–Motor Integration.* Cleveland, OH: Modern Curriculum Press.

Begali, V. (1992). *Head injury in children and adolescents* (2nd ed.). Brandon, VT: Clinical Psychology Publishing.

Benton, A. L., Hamsher, K. deS., Varyney, N. R., & Spreen, O. (1983). *Contributions to neuropsychological assessment: A clinical manual.* New York: Oxford University Press.

Bergland, M. M. (1996). Transition from school to adult life: Key to the future. In A. L. Goldberg (Ed.), *Acquired brain injury in childhood and adolescence* (pp. 171–194). Springfield, IL: Charles C. Thomas.

Berninger, V. W., Abbott, S. P., Greep, K., & Reed, E. (1997). Directed reading and writing activities: Aiming instruction to working brain systems. In S. M. C. Dollinger & L. F. DiLalla (Eds.), *Assessment and intervention issues across the life span* (pp. 123–158). Mahwah, NJ: Erlbaum.

Bigler, E. D., Johnson, S. C., & Blatter, D. D. (1999). Head trauma and intellectual status: Relation to quantitative magnetic resonance imaging findings. *Applied Neuropsychology, 6,* 217–225.

Bijur, P., & Haslum, M. (1995). Cognitive, behavioral, and motoric sequelae of mild head injury in a national birth cohort. In S. H. Broman & M. E. Michel (Eds.), *Traumatic head injury in children* (pp. 147–164). New York: Oxford University Press.

Bijur, P., Haslum, M., & Golding, J. (1990). Cognitive and behavioral sequelae of mild head injury in children. *Pediatrics, 86,* 337–344.

Binder, L. M., & Rattok, J. (1989). Assessment of the postconcussive syndrome after mild head trauma. In M. D. Lezak (Ed.), *Assessment of the behavioral consequences of head trauma* (pp. 37–48). New York: Liss.

Bloom, D., Ewing-Cobbs, L., Fletcher, J., Levin, H., Song, J., & Brookshire, B. (2000). Long-term academic outcome following pediatric traumatic brain injury. *Journal of the International Neuropsychological Society, 6,* 226.

Blosser, J. L., & DePompei, R. (1994). *Pediatric traumatic brain injury: Proactive intervention.* San Diego, CA: Singular.

Boll, T. (1982). Behavioral sequelae of head injury. In P. Cooper (Ed.), *Head injury* (pp. 363–377). Baltimore, MD: Williams & Wilkins.

Boll, T. (1983). Minor head injury in children—Out of sight, but not out of mind. *Journal of Clinical Child Psychology, 12*, 74–80.

Bos, C. S., & Vaughn, S. (1988). *Strategies for teaching students with learning and behavior problems.* Boston: Allyn & Bacon.

Bowden, H. N., Knights, R., & Winogron, H. W. (1985). Speeded performance following head injury in children. *Journal of Clinical and Experimental Neuropsychology, 7*, 39–54.

Braswell, L., & Bloomquist, M. L. (1991). *Cognitive–behavioral therapy with ADHD children: Child, family, and school interventions.* New York: Guilford Press.

Brazelli, B., Colombo, N., Della Sala, S., & Spinnier, H. (1994). Spared and impaired cognitive abilities after bilateral frontal damage. *Cortex, 30*, 27–51.

Breslau, N. (1982). Siblings of disabled children: Birth order and age-spacing effects. *Journal of Abnormal Child Psychology, 10*, 85–96.

Breslau, N. (1983). The psychological study of chronically ill and disabled children: Are healthy siblings appropriate controls? *Journal of Abnormal Child Psychology, 11*, 379–391.

Brodal, P. (1992). *The central nervous system: Structure and function.* New York: Oxford University Press.

Brooks, D. N. (1990). Behavioral and social consequences of severe head injury. In B. Deelman, R. Soan, & A. van Zomeren (Eds.), *Traumatic brain injury: Clinical, social, and rehabilitation aspects* (pp. 77–88). Amsterdam: Swets & Zeitlinger.

Brooks, D. N. (1991). The head-injury family. *Journal of Clinical and Experimental Neuropsychology, 13*, 155–188.

Brooks, D. N., Campsie, L., Symington, C., Beattie, A., & McKinlay, W. (1986). The five-year outcome of severe blunt head injury: A relative's view. *Journal of Neurology, Neurosurgery, and Psychiatry, 49*, 764–800.

Brooks, D. N., Campsie, L., Symington, C., Beattie, A., & McKinlay, W. (1987). The effects of severe-head injury on patient and relatives within seven years of injury. *Journal of Head Trauma Rehabilitation, 2*, 1–13.

Brown, G., Chadwick, O., Shaffer, D., Rutter, M., & Traub, M. (1981). A prospective study of children with head injuries: III. Psychiatric sequelae. *Psychological Medicine, 11*, 1227–1232.

Bruce, D. A. (1990). Scope of the problem—Early assessment and management. In M. Rosenthal, E. R. Griffith, M. R. Bond, & J. D. Miller (Eds.), *Rehabilitation of the adult and child with traumatic brain injury* (2nd ed., pp. 521–538). Philadelphia: Davis.

Calub, C., Burton, J., DeBoskey, D. S., & Hooker, C. (1989). *A cognitive rehabilitation system: Evaluation, treatment, and generalization.* Tampa, FL: DeBoskey and Associates.

Canter, A. S., & Carroll, S. A. (1998). *Helping children at home and school.* Bethesda, MD: NASP.

Carlson, N. R. (1994). *Physiology of behavior* (5th ed.). Boston: Allyn & Bacon.

Carney, J., & Gerring, J. (1990). Return to school following severe closed head injury: A critical phase in pediatric rehabilitation. *Pediatrician, 17*, 222–229.

Carter, R. . R., & Savage, R. C. (1985). Education and the traumatically brain injured: Rights, protections, and responsibilities. *Cognitive Rehabilitation, 3,* 14–17.

Catroppa, C., Anderson, V., & Stargatt, R. (1999). A prospective analysis of the recovery of attention following pediatric head injury. *Journal of the International Neuropsychological Society, 5,* 48–57.

Chadwick, O., Rutter, M., Brown, G., Shaffer, D., & Traub, M. (1981a). A prospective study of children with head injuries: II. Cognitive sequelae. *Psychological Medicine, 11,* 49–61.

Chadwick, O., Rutter, M., Shaffer, D., & Shrout, P. E. (1981b). A prospective study of children with head injuries: IV. Specific cognitive deficits. *Journal of Clinical Neuropsychology, 3,* 101–120.

Chapman, S. B., Culhane, K. A., Levin, H. S., Harward, H., Mendelsohn, D., Ewing-Cobbs, L., Fletcher, J. M., & Bruce, D. (1992). Narrative discourse after closed head injury in children and adolescents. *Brain and Language, 43,* 42–65.

Clark, E. (1996). Children and adolescents with traumatic brain injury: Reintegration challenges in educational settings. *Journal of Learning Disabilities, 29,* 549–560.

Clark, E., Baker, B. K., Gardner, M. K., Pompa, J. L., & Tait, F. V. (1990). Effectiveness of stimulant drug treatment for attention problems. *School Psychology International, 11,* 227–234.

Code of Federal Regulations 34. (July, 1993). *Parts 300 to 399, Education.* Washington, DC: Office of the Federal Register, National Archives and Records Administration.

Cohen, M. D., & Duffner, P. K. (2000). Tumors of the brain and spinal cord including leukemic involvement. In K. F. Swaiman (Ed.), *Pediatric neurology* (3rd ed., pp. 1049–1098). St. Louis, MO: Mosby.

Cohen, S. B. (1986). Educational reintegration and programming for children with head injuries. *Journal of Head Trauma Rehabilitation, 1,* 22–26.

Cohen, S. B. (1991). Adapting educational programs for students with head injuries. *Journal of Head Trauma Rehabilitation, 6,* 56–63.

Cohen, S. B. (1996). Practical guidelines for teachers. In A. L. Goldberg (Ed.), *Acquired brain injury in childhood and adolescence: A team and family guide to educational program development and implementation* (pp. 126–170). Springfield, IL: Charles C. Thomas.

Cohen, S. B., Joyce, C. M., Rhoades, K. W., & Welks, D. M. (1985). Educational programming for head injured students. In M. Ylvisaker (Ed.), *Head injury rehabilitation: Children and adolescents* (pp. 30–53). San Diego: College-Hill Press.

Comings, D. E. (1990). *Tourette syndrome and human behavior.* Durante, CA: Hope Press.

Conoley, J., & Sheridan, S. (1996). Pediatric traumatic brain injury: Challenges and interventions for families. *Journal of Learning Disabilities, 29,* 662–669.

Cook, J., Berrol, S., Harrington, D., Kanter, M., Knight, N., Miller, C., & Silverman, L. (1987). *ABI handbook: Serving students with acquired brain injury in higher education.* California Community College Chancellor's Office, Disabled Students Programs and Services.

Cope, D. N. (1987). Psychopharmocologic considerations in the treatment of traumatic brain injury. *Journal of Head Trauma Rehabilitation, 2,* 2–5.

Corrigan, J. (1995). Substance abuse as a mediating factor in outcome from traumatic brain injury. *Archives of Physical Medicine and Rehabilitation, 76,* 302–309.

Coutts, R. L., Lichstein, L., Bermudez, J. M., Daigle, M., Mann, R., Charbonnel, T. S., Michaud, R., & Williams, C. R. (1987). Treatment assessment of learning disabled children: Is there a role for frequently repeated neuropsychological testing? *Archives of Clinical Neuropsychology, 2,* 237–244.

Dalby, P. R., & Obrzut, J. E. (1991). Epidemiologic characteristics and sequelae of closed head-injured children and adolescents. *Developmental Neuropsychology, 7,* 35–68.

D'Amato, R. C., & Rothlisberg, B. A. (1996). How education should respond to students with traumatic brain injury. *Journal of Learning Disabilities, 29,* 670–683.

Delis, D. C., Kramer, J. H., Kaplan, E., & Ober, B. A. (1994). *California Verbal Learning Test—Children's Version.* San Antonio, TX: Psychological Corporation.

Dempster, F. M. (1988). The spacing effect. A case study in the failure to apply the results of psychological research. *American Psychologist, 43,* 627–634.

Dennis, M. C., & Barnes, M. A. (1990). Knowing the meaning, getting the point, bridging the gap, and carrying the message: Aspects of discourse following closed head injury in childhood and adolescence. *Brain and Language, 39,* 428–446.

Dennis, M., C. Roncardin, Barnes, M. A., Guger, S., & Archibald, J. (2000). Working memory after mild, moderate, or severe childhood head injury. *Journal of the International Neuropsychological Society, 6,* 132.

Dennis, M., Wilkinson, M., Koski, L., & Humphreys, R. P. (1995). Attention deficits in the long term after childhood head injury. In S. Broman & M. E. Michel (Eds.), *Traumatic head injury in children and adolescents* (pp. 165–187). New York: Oxford University Press.

DePompei, R., & Blosser, J. L. (1993). Professional training and development for pediatric rehabilitation. In C. J. Durgin, N. D. Schmidt, & L. J. Fryer (Eds.), *Staff development and clinical intervention in brain injury rehabilitation* (pp. 229–253). Gaithersburg, MD: Aspen Publications.

DePompei, R., & Zarski, J. (1989). Families, head injury, and cognitive–communicative impairments: Issues for family counseling. *Topics in Language Disorders, 9,* 78–89.

Deshler, D. D., Schumacker, J. B., Lenz, B. K., & Ellis, E. (1984). Academic and cognitive interventions for LD adolescents. *Journal of Learning Disabilities, 17,* 170–179.

Dikmen, S., McLean, A., & Temkin, N. (1986). Neuropsychological and psychosocial consequences of minor head injury. *Journal of Neurology, Neurosurgery, and Psychiatry, 40,* 1227–1232.

Di Scala, C., Osberg, J. S., Gans, B. M., Chin, L. J., & Grant, C. C. (1991). Children with traumatic head injury: Morbidity and postacute treatment. *Archives of Physical Medicine and Rehabilitation, 72,* 662–666.

Donders, J. (1992). Premorbid behavior and psychosocial adjustment of children with traumatic brain injury. *Journal of Abnormal Child Psychology, 20,* 233–246.

Donders, J. (1995). Validity of the Kaufman Brief Intelligence Test (K-BIT) in children with traumatic brain injury. *Assessment, 2,* 219–224.

Donders, J. (1996). Cluster subtypes in the WISC-III standardization sample: Analysis of factor index scores. *Psychological Assessment, 8,* 312–318.

Donders, J. (1997). Sensitivity of the WISC-III to injury severity in children with traumatic head injury. *Assessment, 4,* 107–109.

Donders, J., & Warschausky, S. (1996). A structural equation analysis of the WISC-III in children with traumatic head injury. *Child Neuropsychology, 2,* 185–192.

Donders, J., & Warschausky, S. (1997). WISC-III factor index score patterns after traumatic head injury in children. *Child Neuropsychology, 3,* 71–78.

Doronzo, J. F. (1990). Mild head injury. In E. Lehr (Ed.), *Psychological management of traumatic brain injuries in children and adolescents* (pp. 207–224). Rockville, MD: Aspen.

Dyson, L., Edgar, E., & Crnic, K. (1989). Psychological predictors of adjustment by siblings of developmentally disabled children. *American Journal of Mental Retardation, 94,* 292–302.

Eimas, P. D. (1985). Constraints on a model of infant speech perception. In J. Mehler & R. Fox (Eds.), *Neonate cognition: Beyond the blooming buzzing confusion* (pp. 185–197). Hillsdale, NJ: Erlbaum.

Ewing-Cobbs, L., Fletcher, J. M., & Levin, H. S. (1986). Neurobehavioral sequelae following head injury in children: Educational implications. *Journal of Head Trauma Rehabilitation, 1,* 57–65.

Ewing-Cobbs, L., Fletcher, J. M., & Levin, H. S. (1989). Intellectual, motor, and language sequelae following closed head injury in infants and preschoolers. *Journal of Pediatric Psychology, 14,* 531–547.

Ewing-Cobbs, L., Fletcher, J. M., Levin, H. S., Iovino, I., & Miner, M. E. (1998a). Academic achievement and academic placement following traumatic brain injury in children and adolescents: A two-year longitudinal study. *Journal of Clinical and Experimental Neuropsychology, 20,* 769–781.

Ewing-Cobbs, L., Iovino, I., Fletcher, J. M., Miner, M. E., & Levin, H. S. (1991). Academic achievement following traumatic brain injury in children and adolescents. *Journal of Clinical and Experimental Neuropsychology, 13,* 93.

Ewing-Cobbs, L., Landry, S., Steubing, K., Prasad, M., & Leal, F. (2000). Social competence in young children with inflicted or noninflicted traumatic brain injury (TBI). *Journal of the International Neuropsychological Society, 6,* 226.

Ewing-Cobbs, L., Levin, H. S., Eisenberg, H. M., & Fletcher, J. M. (1987). Language functions following closed-head injury in children and adolescents. *Journal of Clinical and Experimental Neuropsychology, 9,* 575–592.

Ewing-Cobbs, L., Prasad, M., Fletcher, J. M., Levin, H. S., Miner, M. E., & Eisenberg, H. M. (1998b). Attention after pediatric traumatic brain injury: A multidimensional assessment. *Child Neuropsychology, 4,* 35–48.

Farmer, J., Clippard, D. S., Luehr-Wiemann, Y., Wright, E., & Owings, S. (1996). Assessing children with traumatic brain injury during rehabilitation: Promoting school and community reentry. *Journal of Learning Disabilities, 29,* 532–548.

Farmer, J., & Peterson, L. (1995). Pediatric traumatic brain injury: Promoting successful school entry. *School Psychology Review, 24,* 230–243.

Federal Register. (1975). *Education for All Handicapped Children Act*; Public Law 94–142.

Federal Register. (1990). *Individuals with Disabilities Education Act*; Public Law 101–476.

Filipek, P., & Blickman, J. G. (1992). Neurodiagnostic laboratory procedures: Neuroimaging techniques. In R. B. David (Ed.), *Pediatric neurology for the clinician* (pp. 301–329). Norwalk, CT: Appleton-Lange.

Filipek, P., Kennedy, D., & Caviness, V. (1992). Neuroimaging in child neuropsychology. In I. Rapin & S. Segalowitz (Eds.), *Child neuropsychology* (pp. 301–329). Amsterdam: Elsevier Science.

Filipek, P., Semrud-Clikeman, M., Steingard, R. J., Renshaw, P. F., Kennedy, D. N., & Biederman, J. (1998). Volumetric MRI analysis comparing attention-deficit hyperactivity disorder and normal controls. *Neurology, 48,* 589–601.

Fletcher, J., Ewing-Cobbs, L., Francis, D. J., & Levin, H. S. (1995). Variability in outcomes after traumatic brain injury in children: A developmental perspective. In S. H. Broman & M. E. Michel (Eds.), *Traumatic head injury in children* (pp. 3–21). New York: Oxford University Press.

Fletcher, J., Ewing-Cobbs, L., Miner, M., Levin, H., & Eisenberg, H. (1990). Behavioral changes after closed head injury in children. *Journal of Consulting and Clinical Psychology, 58,* 93–98.

Fordyce, D. J., Roueche, J. R., & Prigatano, G. P. (1983). Enhanced emotional reaction in chronic head trauma patients. *Journal of Neurology, Neurosurgery, and Psychiatry, 46,* 620–624.

Frankowski, R. F., Annegers, J. F., & Whitman, S. (1985). Epidemiological and descriptive studies: Part I. In D. Becker & J. T. Povlishock (Eds.), *Central nervous system trauma: Status report* (pp. 33–45). Bethesda, MD: National Institutes of Health, National Institute of Neurological and Communicative Disorders and Stroke.

Friedman, A. H. (1983). Head injuries: Initial evaluation and management. *Postgraduate Medicine, 70,* 219–222.

Gaylord, D. (1991). *Transition strategies that work.* St. Paul, MN: Minnesota Department of Education.

Ghez, C. (1993). Voluntary movement. In E. R. Kandel, J. Schwartz, & T. Jessel (Eds.), *Principles of neural science* (3rd ed., pp. 609–625). New York: Elsevier.

Glenn, M. B. (1987). A pharmocological approach to aggressive and disruptive behaviors after traumatic brain injury: Part 1. *Journal of Head Trauma Rehabilitation, 2,* 71–73.

Goldberg, E., & Costa, L. D. (1981). Hemisphere differences in the acquisition and use of descriptive systems. *Brain and Language, 14,* 144–173.

Golden, C. J. (1981). The Luria–Nebraska Children's Battery: Theory and formulation. In G. W. Hynd & J. E. Obrzut (Eds.), *Neuropsychological assessment and the school-age child: Issues and procedures* (pp. 277–302). Orlando, FL: Grune & Stratton.

Golden, C. J. (1989). The Nebraska Neuropsychological Battery. In C. R. Reynolds & E. Fletcher-Janzen (Eds.), *Handbook of clinical child neuropsychology* (pp. 193–204). New York: Plenum Press.

Graham, D. I., Ford, I., Adams, J. H., Doyle, D., Lawrence, A. E., McLellan, D. R., & Ng, H. K. (1989a). Fatal head injury in children. *Clinical Pathology, 42*, 18–23.

Graham, D. I., Ford, I., Adams, J. H., Doyle, D., Teasdale, G. M., Lawrence, A. E., & McLellan, D. R. (1989b). Ischemic brain damage is still common in fatal, nonmissile head injury. *Journal of Neurology, Neursurgery, and Psychiatry 52*, 346–351.

Green, M. L., Foster, M. A., Morris, M., Muir, J. J., & Morris, R. D. (1998). Parent assessment of psychological and behavioral functioning following pediatric acquired brain injury. *Journal of Pediatric Psychology, 23*, 289–299.

Harrington, D. E. (1990). Educational strategies. In M. Rosenthal, E. R. Griffith, M. R. Bond, & J. D. Miller (Eds.), *Rehabilitation of the adult and child with traumatic brain injury* (2nd ed., pp. 476–492). Philadelphia: Davis.

Harris, B., Schwaitzberg, S., Seman, T., & Herrman, C. (1989). The hidden morbidity of pediatric trauma. *Journal of Pediatric Surgery, 24*, 103–106.

Hashimoto, T., Tayama, M., Miyazaki, M., Fuji, E., Harada, M., Miyoshi, H., Tanouchi, M., & Kuroda, Y. (1995). Developmental brain changes investigated with proton magnetic resonance spectroscopy. *Developmental Medicine and Child Neurology, 37*, 398–405.

Henry, P. C., Hauber, R. P., & Rice, M. (1992). Factors associated with closed head injury in a pediatric population. *Journal of Neuroscience Nursing, 24*, 311–316.

Hoffman, N., Donders, J., & Thompson, E. H. (2000). Novel learning abilities after traumatic head injury in children. *Archives of Clinical Neuropsychology, 15*, 47–58.

Holmes, C. B. (1988). *The head-injured college student.* Springfield, IL: Charles C. Thomas.

Howieson, D. B., & Lezak, M. D. (1992). The neuropsychological evaluation. In S. C. Yudofsky & R. E. Hales (Eds.), *The American Psychiatric Press textbook of neuropsychiatry* (2nd ed., pp. 127–150). Washington, DC: American Psychiatric Press.

Hu, X., Wesson, D., Kenney, B., Chipman, H., & Spence, L. (1993). Risk factors for extended disruption of family function after severe injury to a child. *Canadian Medical Association Journal, 149*, 421–427.

Hynd, G. W. (1992). *Neuropsychological assessment in clinical child psychology.* Newbury Park, CA: Sage.

Hynd, G. W., & Semrud-Clikeman, M. (1990). Neuropsychological batteries in assessment of intelligence. In A. S. Kaufman (Ed.), *Assessing adolescent and adult intelligence* (pp. 638–695). Boston: Allyn & Bacon.

Hynd, G. W., & Willis, W. G. (1988). *Pediatric neuropsychology.* Orlando, FL: Grune & Stratton.

Jackson, A., & Haverkamp, D. E. (1991). Family response to traumatic brain injury. *Counseling Psychology Quarterly, 4*, 355–356.

Jaffe, K. M., Brink, J. D., Hays, R. M., & Chorazy, A. J. L. (1990). Specific problems associated with pediatric head injury. In M. Rosenthal, E. R. Griffith, M. R. Bond, & J. D. Miller (Eds.), *Rehabilitation of the adult and child with traumatic brain injury* (2nd ed., pp. 539–557). Philadelphia: Davis.

Jaffe, K. M., Mastrilli, J., Molitor, C. B., & Valko, A. (1985). Physical rehabilitation. In M. Ylvisaker (Ed.), *Head injury rehabilitation: Children and adolescents* (pp. 167–195). San Diego, CA: College-Hill Press.

Jane, J. A., & Rimel, R. W. (1982). Prognosis in head injury. *Clinical Neurosurgery,* *29,* 346–352.

Janus, P. L. (1994). The role of school administration. In R. C. Savage & G. F. Wolcott (Eds.), *Educational dimensions of acquired brain injury* (pp. 345–365. Austin, TX: Pro-Ed.

Janusz, J., Kirkwood, M., Yeates, K. O., Taylor, H. G., Wade, S., Stancin, T., & Drotar, D. (2000). Prevalence and correlates of depressive symptoms following closed-head injuries in children. *Journal of the International Neuropsychological Society, 6,* 226.

Jennett, B., & Teasdale, G. (1981). *Management of head injuries.* Philadelphia: Davis.

Johnson, D. A. (1992). Head injured children and education: A need for greater delineation and understanding. *British Journal of Educational Psychology, 62,* 404–409.

Johnson, D. A., & Roethig-Johnson, K. (1989). Life in the slow lane: Attentional factors after head injury. In D. A. Johnson, D. Uttley, & M. Wyke (Eds.), *Children's head injuries: Who cares?* (pp. 96–110). New York: Taylor & Francis.

Kandel, E. R., Schwartz, J. H., & Jessell, T. M. (Eds.). (1993). *Principles of neural behavior.* New York: Elsevier.

Kaplan, E. (1988). A process approach to neuropsychological assessment. In T. Boll & B. K. Bryant (Eds.), *Clinical neuropsychology and brain function* (pp. 124–167). Washington DC: American Psychological Association.

Karras, D., Newlin, D. B., Franzen, M. D., Golden, C. J., Wilkening, G. M., Rothermel, R. D., & Tramontana, M. J. (1987). Development of factor scales for the Luria–Nebraska Neuropsychological Battery—Children's Revision. *Journal of Clinical Child Psychology, 16,* 19–28.

Katsiyannis, A., & Conderman, G. (1994). Serving individuals with traumatic brain injury. *Remedial and Special Education, 15,* 319–325.

Kaufmann, P. M., Fletcher, J. M., Levin, H. S., Miner, M. E., & Ewing-Cobbs, L. (1993). Attentional disturbance after closed head injury. *Journal of Child Neurology, 8,* 348–353.

Kehle, T. J., Clark, E., & Jenson, W. R. (1996). Interventions for students with traumatic brain injury: Managing behavioral disturbances. *Journal of Learning Disabilities, 29,* 633–642.

Kehle, T. J., Clark, E., Jenson, W. R., & Wampold, B. E. (1986). Effectiveness of self-observation with behavior disordered elementary school children. *School Psychology Review, 15,* 289–295.

Kehle, T. J., & Gonzales, F. (1991). Self-modeling for emotional and social concerns of childhood. In P. W. Dowrick (Ed.), *A practical guide to video in the behavioral sciences* (pp. 221–252). New York: Wiley.

Kelly, D. F. (1995). Alcohol and head injury: An issue revisited. *Journal of Neurotrauma, 12*, 883–890.

Kelly, M. P., Johnson, C. T., Knoller, N., Drubach, D. A., & Winslow, M. M. (1997). Substance abuse, traumatic brain injury, and neuropsychological outcome. *Brain Injury, 11*, 391–402.

Kendall, P. C., & Braswell, L. (1993). *Cognitive-behavioral therapy for impulsive children* (2nd ed.). New York: Guilford Press.

Kerns, K. A., Thomson, J., & Youngman, P. (1993, March). *Development of a compensatory memory system for an adolescent.* Paper presented at the Pediatric Brain Injury Conference, Vancouver, BC.

Klonoff, H., Low, M. D., & Clark, C. (1977). Head injuries in children: A prospective five-year follow-up. *Journal of Neurology, Neurosurgery, and Psychiatry, 40*, 1211–1215.

Kolb, B., & Fantie, B. (1989). Development of the child's brain and behavior. C. R. Reynolds & E. F. Janzen (Eds.), *Handbook of clinical child neuropsychology* (pp. 17–40). New York: Plenum Press.

Kolb, B., & Whishaw, I. Q. (1990). *Fundamentals of human neuropsychology* (3rd ed.). San Francisco: Freeman.

Kovacs, M. (1992). *Children's Depression Inventory manual.* North Tonawanda, NY: Multi-Health Systems.

Kratochwill, T. R., & Bergan, J. R. (1990). *Behavioral consultation in applied settings: An individual guide.* New York: Plenum Press.

Kraus, J. F. (1995). Epidemiological features of brain injury in children: Occurrence, children at risk, causes and manner of injury, severity, and outcomes. In S. H. Broman & M. E. Michel (Eds.), *Traumatic head injury in children* (pp. 22–39). New York: Oxford University Press.

Kraus, J. F., Rock, A., & Hemyarai, P. (1990). Brain injuries among infants, children, adolescents, and young adults. *American Journal of Diseases of Children, 144*, 684–691.

Kreutzer, J. S., Witol, A. D., Marwitz, J. H. (1996). Alcohol and drug use among young persons with traumatic brain injury. *Journal of Learning Disabilities, 29*, 643–651.

Kupferman, I. (1991). Learning and memory. In E. R. Kandel, J. H. Schwartz, & T. M. Jessel (Eds.), *Principles of neural science* (3rd ed., pp. 997–1008). New York: Elsevier.

Lachar, D., Kline, R. B., & Boersma, D. C. (1986). The Personality Inventory for Children: Approaches to actuarial interpretation in clinic and school settings. In H. M. Knoff (Ed.), *The assessment of child and adolescent personality* (pp. 273–308). New York: Guilford Press.

Lehr, E. (1990). *Psychological management of traumatic brain injuries in children and adolescents.* Rockville, MD: Aspen.

Levi, R. B., Drotar, D., Yeates, K. O., & Taylor, H. G. (1999). Posttraumatic stress symptoms in children following orthopedic or traumatic brain injury. *Journal of Child Clinical Psychology, 28*, 232–243.

Levin, H. S. (1987). Neurobehavioral sequelae of head injury. In P. R. Cooper (Ed.), *Head injury* (2nd ed., pp. 3–27). Baltimore: Williams & Wilkins.

Levin, H. S., Benton, A. L., & Grossman, R. G. (1982). *Neurobehavioral consequences of closed head injury.* New York: Oxford University Press.

Levin, H. S., Culhane, K. A., Fletcher, J. M., & Mendelsohn, D. B. (1994). Dissociation between delayed attention and memory after pediatric head injury: Relationship to MRI findings. *Journal of Child Neurology, 9,* 81–89.

Levin, H. S., Culhane, K. A., Lilly, M. A., Bruce, D., Fletcher, J. M., Chapman, S. B., Harward, H., & Eisenberg, H. M. (1993). Cognition in relation to magnetic resonance imaging in head-injured children and adolescents. *Archives of Neurology, 50,* 897–905.

Levin, H. S., & Eisenberg, H. M. (1979). Neuropsychological impairment after closed head injury in children and adolescents. *Journal of Pediatric Psychology, 4,* 389–402.

Levin, H. S., Ewing-Cobbs, L., & Eisenberg, H. M. (1995). Neurobehavioral outcome of pediatric closed head injury. In S. Broman & M. E. Michel (Eds.), *Traumatic head injury in children* (pp. 70–94). New York: Oxford University Press.

Levin, H. S., Fletcher, J. M., Kusnerik, L., & Kufera, J. A. (1996). Semantic memory following pediatric head injury: Relationship to age, severity of injury, and MRI. *Cortex, 32,* 461–478.

Levin, H. S., High, W. M., Jr., Ewing-Cobbs, L., Fletcher, J. M., Eisenberg, H. M., Miner, M. E., & Goldstein, F. C. (1988). Memory functioning during the first year after closed head injury in children and adolescents. *Neurosurgery, 22,* 1043–1052.

Lewis, R. D., Hutchens, T. A., & Garland, B. L. (1993). Cross-validation of the discriminative effectiveness of the Luria–Nebraska Neuropsychological Battery for learning disabled adolescents. *Archives of Clinical Neuropsychology, 8,* 437–447.

Lezak, M. (1988). Brain damage is a family affair. *Journal of Clinical and Experimental Neuropsychology, 10,* 111–123.

Lezak, M. (1994). *Neuropsychological assessment* (4th ed.). New York: Oxford University Press.

Lindamood, C. H., & Lindamood, P. (1998). *Auditory Discrimination in Depth.* Austin, TX: Pro-Ed.

Lockman, L. A. (1994). Nonabsence generalized seizures. In K. F. Swaiman (Ed.), *Pediatric neurology* (2nd ed., pp. 261–270). St. Louis, MO: Mosby.

Lord-Maes, J., & Obrzut, J. E. (1996). Neuropsychological consequences of traumatic brain injury in children and adolescents. *Journal of Learning Disabilities, 29,* 609–617.

Luerssen, T. G., Klauber, M. R., & Marshall, L. F. (1988). Outcome from head injury related to patient's age: A longitudinal prospective study of adult and pediatric head injury. *Journal of Neurosurgery, 68,* 409–416.

Luria, A. R. (1963). *Restoration of function after brain injury.* New York: Macmillan.

Luria, A. R. (1980). *Higher cortical functions in man* (2nd ed.). New York: Basic Books.

Lustig, A. P., & Tompkins, C. A. (1998). An examination of severity classification measures and subject criteria used for studies on mild pediatric traumatic brain injury. *Journal of Medical Speech-Language Pathology, 6,* 13–25.

Mahalick, D. M. (1990). *The neuropsychological sequelae of arteriovenous malformations.* Unpublished dissertation, California School of Professional Psychology, San Diego, CA.

Mapou, R. L. (1992). Neuropathology and neuropsychology of behavioral disturbance following traumatic brain injury. In C. L. Long & L. K. Ross (Eds.), *Handbook of head trauma: Acute care to recovery* (pp. 75–90). New York: Plenum Press.

Martin, D. A. (1988). Children and adolescents with traumatic brain injury: Impact on the family. *Journal of Learning Disabilities, 21,* 464–470.

Martin, R. C. (1993). Short-term memory and sentence processing: Evidence from neuropsychology. *Memory and Cognition, 21,* 176–183.

Mateer, C. A., Kerns, K. A., & Eso, K. L. (1996). Management of attention and memory disorders following traumatic brain injury. *Journal of Learning Disabilities, 29,* 618–632.

Mauss-Clum, N., & Ryan, N. (1981). Brain injury and the family. *Journal of Neurosurgical Nurses, 13,* 165–169.

McAllister, T. W. (1992). Neuropsychiatric sequelae of head injuries. *Psychiatric Clinics of North America, 15,* 522–534.

McKee, W. T., & Witt, J. C. (1990). Effective teaching: A review of instructional and environmental variables. In T. B. Gutkin & C. R. Reynolds (Eds.), *The handbook of school psychology* (pp. 821–846). New York: Wiley.

McKinlay, W. W., Brooks, M. R., Bond, M. R., Martinage, D. P., & Marshall, M. M. (1981). The short-term outcome of severe blunt head injury as reported by relatives of the injured patients. *Journal of Neurology, Neurosurgery, and Psychiatry, 48,* 527–533.

Mendelsohn, D., Levin, H. S., Bruce, D. A., Lilly, M., Harward, H., Culhane, K. A., & Eisenberg, H. M. (1992). Later MRI after head injury in children: Relationship to clinical features and outcome. *Child Nervous System, 8,* 445–452.

Mercer, C. D., & Mercer, A. R. (1989). *Teaching students with learning problems.* Columbus, OH: Merrill.

Michaud, L. J. (1995). Evaluating efficacy of rehabilitation after pediatric traumatic brain injury. In S. H. Broman and M. E. Michel (Eds.), *Traumatic head injury in children* (pp. 247–257). New York: Oxford University Press.

Michaud, L. J., Duhaime, A., & Batshaw, M. L. (1993). Traumatic brain injury in children. *Pediatric Clinics of North America, 40,* 553–565.

Midgley, C., Feldaufer, H., & Eccles, J. S. (1989). Change in teacher efficacy and student self- and task-related beliefs in mathematics during the transition from junior high school. *Journal of Educational Psychology, 81,* 247–258.

Milberg, W. B., Hebben, N., & Kaplan, E. (1986). The Boston Process Approach to neuropsychological assessment. In I. Grant & K. M. Adams (Eds.), *Neuropsychological assessment and neuropsychiatric disorders* (pp. 65–86). New York: Oxford University Press.

Miller, L. (1993). Family therapy of brain injury: Syndromes, strategies, and solutions. *The American Journal of Family Therapy, 21,* 111–121.

Mira, M. P., & Tyler, J. S. (1991). Students with traumatic brain injury: Making the transition from hospital to school. *Focus on Exceptional Children, 23*, 1–12.

Mittenberg, W., Wittner, M. S., & Miller, L. J. (1997). Postconcussion syndrome occurs in children. *Neuropsychology, 11*, 447–452.

Molfese, D. L., & Molfese, V. J. (1986). Psychophysiological indices of early cognitive processes and their relationship to language. In J. E. Obrzut & G. W. Hynd (Eds.), *Child neuropsychology: Theory and research* (pp. 95–115). New York: Academic Press.

Nass, R., Peterson, H., & Koch, D. (1989). Differential effects of congenital left and right brain injury on intelligence. *Brain and Cognition, 9*, 258–266.

National Head Injury Foundation. (1985). *An educator's manual: What educators need to know about students with traumatic head injury*. Framingham, MA: Author.

National Institutes of Health. (1998). Rehabilitation of persons with traumatic brain injury. *National Institutes of Health Consensus Statement, 16*, 1–41.

National Joint Committee on Learning Disabilities. (1992). School reform: Opportunities for excellence and equity for individuals with learning disabilities. *Journal of Learning Disabilities, 25*, 276–280.

Naugle, R. (1990). Epidemiology of traumatic brain injury in adults. In E. D. Bigler (Ed.), *Traumatic brain injury: Mechanisms of damage, assessment, intervention, and outcome* (pp. 69–103). Austin, TX: Pro-Ed.

Newton, M. R., Greenwood, R. J., Britton, K. E., Charlesworth, M., Nimmon, C. C., Carroll, M. J., & Dolke, G. (1992). A study comparing SPECT with CT and MRI after closed head injury. *Journal of Neurology, Neurosurgery, and Psychiatry, 55*, 92–100.

Nichols, S., Jones, W., Delis, D. C., Wulfeck, B., & Trauner, D. (2000). The effects of early focal brain injury on verbal learning and memory. *Journal of the International Neuropsychological Society, 6*, 131.

O'Leary, D. S., & Boll, T. J. (1984). Neuropsychological correlates of early generalized brain dysfunction in children. In C. R. Almli & S. Finger (Eds.), *Early brain damage: Vol. 1. Research orientations and clinical observations*. Orlando, FL: Academic Press.

Orsillo, S. M., McCaffrey, R. J., & Fisher, J. M. (1993). Siblings of head-injured individuals: A population at risk. *Journal of Head Trauma Rehabilitation, 8*, 102–115.

Ozer, M. (1988). *The head injury survivor on campus: Issues and resources*. Washington, DC: Health Resource Center.

Pang, D. (1985). Pathophysiologic correlations of neurobehavioral syndromes following closed head injury. In M. Ylvisaker (Ed.), *Head injury rehabilitation: Children and adolescents* (pp. 3–71). San Diego: College-Hill Press.

Papas, B. (1993). Managing aggression: New strategies for the hospital setting. *Headlines, 4*, 2–8.

Pennington, B. F. (1991). *Diagnosing learning disorders: A neuropsychological approach*. New York: Guilford Press.

Perrott, S., Taylor, H., & Montes, J. (1991). Neuropsychological sequelae, family stress, and environmental adaptation following pediatric head injury. *Developmental Neuropsychology, 7*, 69–86.

Posner, M. I., & Raichle, M. E. (1994). *Images of mind.* New York: Scientific American Library.

Prasad, M., Ewing-Cobbs, L., Landry, S., & Kramer, L. (2000). Premorbid child characteristics and recovery from traumatic brain injury in infants and pre-schoolers. *Journal of the International Neuropsychological Society, 6,* 226.

Prigatano, G. P. (1985). *Neuropsychological rehabilitation after brain injury.* Baltimore, MD: Johns Hopkins Press.

Prigatano, G. P. (2000). Principles of neuropsychological rehabilitation in the year 2000. *Brain Injury Source, 4,* 20–21.

Raimondi, A. J., & Hirschauer, J. (1984). Head injury in the infant and toddler: Coma scoring and outcome scale. *Child's Brain, 11,* 12–35.

Rayport, S. G. (1992). Cellular and molecular biology of the neuron. In S. C. Yudofsky & R. E. Hales (Eds.), *The American Psychiatric Press textbook of neuropsychiatry* (2nd ed., pp. 3–28). Washington, DC: American Psychiatric Press.

Reavis, H. K., Jenson, W. R., Kukic, S. J., & Morgan, D. P. (1993). *Utah's BEST project: Behavioral and educational strategies for teachers.* Salt Lake City: Utah State Office of Education.

Reid, D., & Kelly, M. (1993). Wechsler Memory Scale—Revised in closed head injury. *Journal of Clinical Psychology, 49,* 245–253.

Reitan, R. M., & Wolfson, D. (1985a). *The Halstead–Reitan Neuropsychological Battery: Theory and clinical interpretation.* Tucson, AZ: Neuropsychology Press.

Reitan, R. M., & Wolfson, D. (1985b). *Neuroanatomy and neuropathology: A clinical guide for neuropsychologists.* Tucson, AZ: Neuropsychology Press.

Reynolds, C. R., & Richmond, B. O. (1978). What I Think and Feel: A revised measure of children's manifest anxiety. *Journal of Abnormal Child Psychology, 6,* 271–280.

Rhode, G., Jenson, W. R., & Reavis, H. K. (1993). *The tough kid book: Practical classroom management strategies.* Longmont, CO: Sopris West.

Richards, R. (1998). *The writing dilemma: Understanding dysgraphia.* Riverside, CA: RET Center Press.

Rimel, R., Giordani, B., Barth, J., & Jane, J. (1982). Moderate head injury: Completing the clinical spectrum of brain trauma. *Neurosurgery, 11,* 344–351.

Rivara, J., Fay, G., Jaffe, K., Polissar, N., Shurtleff, H., & Martin, K. (1992). Predictors of family functioning one year following traumatic brain injury in children. *Archives of Physical Medicine Rehabilitation, 73,* 899–910.

Rivara, J., Jaffe, K., Fay, G., Polisser, N., Martin, K., Shurtleff, H., & Liao, S. (1993). Family functioning and injury severity as predictors of child functioning one year following traumatic brain injury. *Archives of Physical Medicine Rehabilitation, 74,* 1047–1055.

Roman, M. J., Delis, D. C., Willerman, L., Magulac, M., Demadura, T. L., de la Pena, J. L., Loftis, C., Walsh, J., & Kracun, M. (1998). Impact of pediatric traumatic brain injury on components of verbal memory. *Journal of Clinical and Experimental Neuropsychology, 20,* 245–258.

Rose, M. J. (1988). The place of drugs in the management of behavior disorders after traumatic brain injury. *Journal of Head Trauma Rehabilitation, 3,* 7–13.

Rosen, C. D., & Gerring, J. P. (1986). *Head trauma educational reintegration.* San Diego, CA: College-Hill Press.

Rosenthal, M., & Bond, M. R. (1990). Behavioral and psychiatric sequelae. In M. Rosenthal, M. Bond, E. R. Griffith, & J. D. Miller (Eds.), *Rehabilitation of the adult and child with traumatic brain injury* (pp. 179–192). Philadelphia: Davis.

Rosenthal, M., & Muir, C. A. (1983). Methods of family intervention. In M. Rosenthal, E. R. Griffith, & M. R. Bond (Eds.), *Rehabilitation of the head injured adult* (pp. 407–419). Philadelphia: Davis.

Rosner, S. L., Abrams, J. C., Daniels, P. R., & Schiffman, G. B. (1981). Dealing with the reading needs of the learning disabled child. *Journal of Learning Disabilities, 14,* 436–448.

Rourke, B. P., Bakker, D. J., Fisk, J. L., & Strang, J. D. (1983). *Child neuropsychology: An introduction to theory, research, and clinical practice.* New York: Guilford Press.

Ruff, R. M., Marshall, L. F., Klauber, M. R., Blunt, B. A., Grant, I., Foulkes, M. A., Eisenberg, H., Jane, J., & Marmarou, A. (1990). Alcohol abuse and neuropsychological outcome of the severely head injured. *Journal of Head Trauma Rehabilitation, 5,* 21–31.

Ruff, R. M., Wylie, T., & Tennant, W. (1993). Malingering and malingering-like aspects of mild closed head injury. *Journal of Head Trauma Rehabilitation, 8,* 60–73.

Ruijs, M. B. M., Keyser, A., & Gabreels, F. J. M. (1990). Long-term sequelae of brain damage from closed head injury in children and adolescents. *Clinical Neurology and Neurosurgery, 92,* 323–328.

Russell, N. K. (1993). Educational considerations in traumatic brain injury: The role of the speech/language pathologist. *Language, Speech, and Hearing Services in Schools, 24,* 67–75.

Rutter, M. (1981). Psychological sequelae of brain damage in children. *American Journal of Psychiatry, 138,* 12–18.

Rutter, M., Chadwick, O., & Shaffer, D. (1983). Head injury. In M. Rutter (Ed.), *Developmental neuropsychiatry* (pp. 83–111). New York: Guilford Press.

Sagvolden, T., & Archer, T. (1989). *Attention deficit disorder: Clinical and basic research.* Hillsdale, NJ: Erlbaum.

Sattler, J. (1990). *Assessment of Children.* San Diego: Author.

Savage, R. C. (1991). Identification, classification, and placement issues for students with traumatic brain injuries. *Journal of Head Trauma Rehabilitation, 6,* 1–9.

Savage, R. C., & Wolcott, G. F. (1988). *An educator's manual: What educators need to know about students with traumatic brain injury.* Southborough, MA: National Head Injury Foundation, Special Education Task Force.

Scheibel, A. B. (1990). Dendritic correlates of higher cognitive function. In A. B. Scheibel & A. F. Wechsler (Eds.), *Neurobiology of higher cognitive function* (pp. 239–270). New York: Guilford Press.

Semrud-Clikeman, M. (1995). *Child and adolescent therapy.* Boston: Allyn & Bacon.

Semrud-Clikeman, M. (1999). Psychosocial aspects of neurological impairments in children. In V. Schwean & D. Sakolfske (Eds.), *Handbook of psychosocial characteristics of exceptional children* (pp. 299–328). New York: Plenum Press.

Semrud-Clikeman, M., Bennett, L., & Guli, L. (in press). Childhood depression. In C. R. Reynolds & R. W. Kamphaus (Eds.), *Handbook of psychological and educational assessment of children* (2nd ed.). New York: Guilford Press.

Semrud-Clikeman, M., & Griffin, J. (2000). Review of cognitive neuroscience. *School Psychology Quarterly, 15,* 105–110.

Semrud-Clikeman, M., & Hynd, G. W. (1990). Right hemispheric dysfunction in nonverbal learning disabilities: Social, academic, and adaptive function in adults and children. *Psychological Bulletin, 107,* 196–207.

Semrud-Clikeman, M., & Hynd, G. W. (1991). Specific nonverbal and social skills deficits in children with learning disabilities. In J. E. Obrzut & G. W. Hynd (Eds.), *Neuropsychological foundations of learning disabilities: A handbook of issues, methods, and practice* (pp. 603–630). San Diego: Academic Press.

Semrud-Clikeman, M., Harrington, K., Parle, N., Clinton, A., & Connor, R. (1999). Innovative interventions with children with attentional difficulties in the school setting. *Journal of Learning Disabilities, 32,* 581–590.

Semrud-Clikeman, M., Steingard, R., Filipek, P. A., Bekken, K., Biederman, J., & Renshaw, P. (2000). Neuroanatomical–neuropsychological correlates of ADHD. *Journal of the American Academy of Child and Adolescent Psychiatry, 39,* 477–484.

Semrud-Clikeman, M., & Wical, B. (1999). Components of attention and memory in complex-partial epilepsy in children with and without ADHD. *Epilepsia, 40,* 211–215.

Shaffer, D. (1995). Behavioral sequelae of serious head injury in children and adolescents: The British studies. In S. H. Broman & M. E. Michel (Eds.), *Traumatic head injury in children* (pp. 55–69). New York: Oxford University Press.

Shapiro, E. S. (1996). *Academic skills problems: Direct assessment and intervention* (2nd ed.). New York: Guilford Press.

Shepard, G. M. (1994). *Neurobiology* (3rd ed.). New York: Oxford University Press.

Sheridan, S., Kratochwill, T. R., & Bergan, J. R. (1996). *Conjoint behavioral consultation: A procedural manual.* New York: Plenum Press.

Shurtleff, H. A., Gay, G. E., Abbott, R. D., & Berninger, V. W. (1988). Cognitive and neuropsychological correlates of academic achievement: A levels of analysis assessment model. *Journal of Psychoeducational Assessment, 6,* 298–308.

Silver, J. M., & Yudofsky, S. C. (1987). Aggressive behavior in patients with neuropsychiatric disorders. *Psychiatric Annals, 17,* 367–370.

Silver, L. B. (1991). The regular education initiative: A déjà vu remembered with sadness and concern. *Journal of Learning Disabilities, 24,* 551–558.

Simeonsson, R. J., & Bailey, D. B. (1986). Siblings of handicapped children. In J. J. Gallagher & P. M. Vietze (Eds.), *Families of handicapped persons: Research, programs and policy issues* (pp. 67–77). Baltimore: Brookes.

Smith, C. R. (1991). *Learning disabilities: The interaction of learner, task, and setting* (2nd ed.). Boston: Allyn & Bacon.

Sohlberg, M. M., & Mateer, C. A. (1987). Effects of an attention training program. *Journal of Clinical and Experimental Neuropsychology, 19,* 117–130.

Sohlberg, M. M., & Mateer, C. A. (1989a). *Introduction to cognitive rehabilitation: Theory and practice.* New York: Guilford Press.

Sohlberg, M. M., & Mateer, C. A. (1989b). Training use of compensatory memory books: A three stage behavioral approach. *Journal of Clinical and Experimental Neuropsychology, 11,* 871–891.

Swaiman, K. F. (1994a). *Pediatric neurology.* St. Louis, MO: Mosby.

Swaiman, K. F. (1994b). Cerebellar dysfunction and ataxia in childhood. In K. F. Swaiman (Ed.), *Pediatric neurology* (2nd ed., pp. 261–270). St. Louis, MO: Mosby.

Tallal, P., Miller, S., Bedi, G., Wang, X., & Nagarajan, S. S. (1996). Language comprehension in language-learning impaired children improved with acoustically modified speech. *Science, 271,* 81–84.

Taylor, H. G., Drotar, D., Wade, S., Yeates, K., Stancin, T., & Klein, S. (1995). Recovery from traumatic brain injury in children: The importance of the family. In S. Broman & M. E. Michel (Eds.), *Traumatic head injury in children* (pp. 188–216). New York: Oxford University Press.

Taylor, H. G., Fletcher, J. M., & Satz, P. (1984). Neuropsychological assessment of children. In G. Goldstein & M. Hersen (Eds.), *Handbook of psychological assessment.* New York: Pergamon Press.

Teeter, P. A. (1986). Standard neuropsychological batteries for children. In J. E. Obrzut & G. W. Hynd (Eds.), *Child neuropsychology: Clinical practice* (pp. 187–228). Orlando, FL: Academic Press.

Teeter, P. A. (1998). *Interventions for ADHD: Treatment in developmental context.* New York: Guilford Press.

Teeter, P. A., & Semrud-Clikeman, M. (1997). *Child neuropsychology: Assessment and interventions for neurodevelopmental disorders.* Boston: Allyn & Bacon.

Teeter, P. A., Uphoff, C. A., Obzrut, J. E., & Malsch, K. (1986). Diagnostic utility of the critical level formula and clinical summary scales of the Luria–Nebraska Neuropsychological Battery—Children's Revision with learning disabled children. *Developmental Neuropsychology, 2,* 125–135.

Telzrow, C. F. (1987). Management of academic and educational problems in head injury. *Journal of Learning Disabilities, 20,* 536–545.

Thatcher, R. W. (1991). Maturation of the human frontal lobes: Physiological evidence for staging. *Developmental Psychology, 7,* 397–419.

Thatcher, R. W. (1994). Cyclic cortical reorganization: Origins of human cognitive development. In G. Dawson & K. W. Fischer (Eds.), *Human behavior and the developing brain* (pp. 232–266). New York: Guilford Press.

Thompson, N. M., Francis, D. J., Steubing, K. K., & Fletcher, J. M. (1994). Motor, visual spatial, and somatosensory skills after closed head injury in children and adolescents: A study of change. *Neuropsychology, 8,* 333–342.

Thomsen, I. V. (1984). Late outcome of very severe blunt head trauma: A 10–15 year second follow-up. *Journal of Neurology, Neurosurgery, and Psychiatry, 47,* 260–268.

Thomson, J. (1995). Rehabilitation of high school-aged individuals with traumatic brain injury through utilization of an attention training program. *Journal of the International Neuropsychological Society, 1,* 149.

Thomson, J., & Kerns, K. A. (in press). Cognitive rehabilitation of the child with mild traumatic brain injury. In S. Raskin & C. A. Mateer (Eds.), *Neuropsychological management of mild traumatic brain injury.* New York: Oxford University Press.

Tompkins, C. A., Holland, A. L., Ratcliff, G., & Costello, A. J. (1990). Predicting cognitive recovery from closed head injury in children and adolescents. *Brain and Cognition, 13,* 86–97.

Tramontana, M., Hooper, S., & Nardillo, E. M. (1988). Behavioral manifestations of neuropsychological impairment in children with psychiatric disorders. *Archives of Clinical Neuropsychology, 3,* 369–374.

Tranel, D. (1992). Functional neuroanatomy: Neuropsychological correlates of cortical and subcortical damage. In S. C. Yudofsky & R. E. Hales (Eds.), *The American Psychiatric Press textbook of neuropsychiatry* (2nd ed., pp. 57–88). Washington, DC: American Psychiatric Press.

Tysvaer, A. (1992). Head and neck injuries in soccer: Impact of minor trauma. *Sports Medicine, 14,* 200–213.

Tysvaer, A., Storli, O. V., & Bachen, N. I. (1989). Soccer injuries to the brain: A neurologic and electroencephalographic study of former players. *Acta-Neurology Scandanavia, 80,* 151–156.

Van Zomeren, A. H., & Brouwer, W. H. (1992). Assessment of attention. In J. R. Crawford, D. M. Parker, & W. W. McKinlay (Eds.), *A handbook of neuropsychological assessment* (pp. 241–266). Hillsdale, NJ: Erlbaum.

Vriezen, E. R. (2000). Cognitive and behavioral sequelae of very mild head injury in children. *Journal of the International Neuropsychological Society, 6,* 131.

Vygotsky, L. S. (1993). *The collected works of L. S. Vygotsky.* New York: Plenum Press.

Waaland, P., Burns, C., & Cockrell, J. (1993). Evaluation of needs of high-and low-income families following pediatric traumatic brain injury. *Brain Injury, 7,* 135–146.

Waaland, P., & Kreutzer, J. (1991). Family response to childhood traumatic brain injury. *Journal of Head Trauma Rehabilitation, 3,* 51–63.

Wade, S., Drotar, D., Taylor, H. G., & Stancin, T. (1995). Assessing the effects of traumatic brain injury on family functioning: Conceptual and methodological issues. *Journal of Pediatric Psychology, 20,* 737–752.

Wade, S., Taylor, H. G., Drotar, D., Stancin, T., & Yeates, K. O. (1996). Childhood traumatic brain injury: Initial impact on the family. *Journal of Learning Disabilities, 29,* 652–661.

Wagstyl, J., Sutcliffe, A. J., & Alpar, E. K. (1987). Early prediction of outcome following head injury in children. *Journal of Pediatric Surgery, 22,* 127–129.

Walker, N., William, B., & Cobb, H. (1999). Training of school psychologists in neuropsychology and brain injury: Results of a national survey of training programs. *Child Neuropsychology, 5,* 137–142.

Wechsler, D. (1991). *Wechsler Intelligence Scale for Cchildren—III.* San Antonio, TX: Psychological Corporation.

Wehman, P. (1992). *Life beyond the classroom: Transition strategies for young people with disabilities.* Baltimore: Brookes.

Weinstein, C. E. (1994). Learning strategies and learning to learn. In *Encyclopedia of education.* New York: Philosophical Library.

West, M., Kregel, J., & Wehman, P. (1991). Assisting young adults with severe TBI to get and keep employment through a supported work approach. *OSERS: News in Print, 4,* 25–30.

Wilens, T. E. (1999). *Straight talk about psychiatric medications for kids.* New York: Guilford Press.

Wilkinson, J. L. (1986). *Neuroanatomy for medical students.* Bristol, England: John Wright & Son, Ltd.

Williams, D. J. (1989). *A process-specific training program in the treatment of attention deficits in children.* Unpublished doctoral dissertation, University of Washington, Seattle.

Willis, W. G., & Widerstrom, A. H. (1986). Structure and function in prenatal and postnatal neuropsychologicl development: A dynamic interaction. In J. E. Obzrut & G. W. Hynd (Eds.), *Child neuropsychology: Theory and research* (pp. 13–53). Orlando, FL; Academic Press.

Wilson, B. A., & Moffat, N. (1984). *Clinical management of memory problems.* Rockville, MD: Aspen.

Winogron, H. W., Knights, R. M., & Bowden, H. N. (1984). Neuropsychological deficits following head injury in children. *Journal of Clinical Neuropsychology, 6,* 269–286.

Witol, A., & Webbe, F. (1994). Neuropsychological deficits associated with soccer play. *Archives of Clinical Neuropsychology, 9,* 204–205.

Wood, R. L. (1987). *Brain injury rehabilitation: A neurobehavioral approach.* Rockville, MD: Aspen.

Woolfolk, A. (2001). *Educational psychology.* Boston: Allyn & Bacon.

Woolsey, C. N. (1958). Organization of somatic and motor areas of the cerebral cortex. In H. F. Harlow & C. N. Woolsey (Eds.), *Biological and biochemical bases of behavior* (pp. 63–81). Madison, WI: University of Wisconsin.

Yeates, K. O., Blumenstein, E., Patterson, E. M., & Delis, D. C. (1995). Verbal learning and memory following pediatric closed-head injury. *Journal of the International Neuropsychological Society, 1,* 78–87.

Yeates, K. O., & Taylor, H. G. (1997). Predicting premorbid neuropsychological functioning following pediatric traumatic brain injury. *Journal of Clinical and Experimental Neuropsychology, 19,* 825–837.

Ylvisaker, M. (1985). *Head injury rehabilitation: Children and adolescents.* San Diego: College-Hill Press.

Ylvisaker, M. (1986). Language and communication disorders following pediatric head injury. *Journal of Head Trauma Rehabilitation, 1,* 48–56.

Ylvisaker, M. (1993). Communication outcome in children and adolescents with traumatic brain injury. *Neuropsychological Rehabilitation, 3,* 367–387.

Ylvisaker, M. (1998). Language and communication disorders following pediatric head injury. *Journal of Head Trauma Rehabilitation, 1,* 48–56.

Ylvisaker, M., Chorazy, A. J. L., Cohen, S. B., Mastrilli, J. P., Molitor, C. B., Nelson,

J., Szekeres, S. F., Valko, A. S., & Jaffe, K. M. (1990). Rehabilitative assessment following head injury in children. In M. Rosenthal, E. R. Griffith, M. R. Bond, & J. D. Miller (Eds.), *Rehabilitation of the adult and child with traumatic brain injury* (2nd ed., pp. 558–592). Philadelphia: Davis.

Ylvisaker, M., Feeney, T. J., & Urbanczyk, B. (1993). A social–environmental approach to communication and behavior after traumatic brain injury. *Seminars in Speech and Language, 14*, 74–87.

Zaidel, E., Clark, M., & Suyenobu, B. (1990). Hemispheric independence: A paradigm case for cognitive neuroscience. In A. B. Scheibel & A. F. Wechsler (Eds.), *Neurobiology of higher cognitive function* (pp. 297–356). New York: Guilford Press.

Index

♦